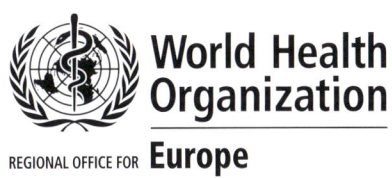

European action plan to reduce the harmful use of alcohol 2012–2020

Keywords
ALCOHOL DRINKING – adverse effects
ALCOHOLISM – prevention and control
ALCOHOLISM AND DRUG ABUSE
HARM REDUCTION
HEALTH EDUCATION
HEALTH POLICY

ISBN 978 92 890 0286 8
Images: Coverpage: GettyImage.com. Page VI, 1, 2, 3, 4, 5, 7, 8, 9, 11, 12, 13, 15, 17, 18, 19, 20, 22, 24, 25, 26, 28, 29, 30, 31, 36, 38, 42, 72: Colourbox.dk. Page 32, 34: Multimedia.euro.who.int.

Address requests about publications of the WHO Regional Office for Europe to:
  Publications
  WHO Regional Office for Europe
  Scherfigsvej 8
  DK–2100 Copenhagen Ø, Denmark
Alternatively, complete an online request form for documentation, health information, or for permission to quote or translate, on the Regional Office web site (http://www.euro.who.int/pubrequest).

© **World Health Organization 2012**

All rights reserved. The Regional Office for Europe of the World Health Organization welcomes requests for permission to reproduce or translate its publications, in part or in full.

The designations employed and the presentation of the material in this publication do not imply the expression of any opinion whatsoever on the part of the World Health Organization concerning the legal status of any country, territory, city or area or of its authorities, or concerning the delimitation of its frontiers or boundaries. Dotted lines on maps represent approximate border lines for which there may not yet be full agreement.

The mention of specific companies or of certain manufacturers' products does not imply that they are endorsed or recommended by the World Health Organization in preference to others of a similar nature that are not mentioned. Errors and omissions excepted, the names of proprietary products are distinguished by initial capital letters.

All reasonable precautions have been taken by the World Health Organization to verify the information contained in this publication. However, the published material is being distributed without warranty of any kind, either express or implied. The responsibility for the interpretation and use of the material lies with the reader. In no event shall the World Health Organization be liable for damages arising from its use. The views expressed by authors, editors, or expert groups do not necessarily represent the decisions or the stated policy of the World Health Organization.

Contents

Foreword V

The European action plan to reduce the harmful use of alcohol 2012–2020 1

    The need for strengthened action in Europe 1

    Policy response in Europe 4

Ten action areas 9

    Leadership, awareness and commitment 9

    Health services' response 12

    Community and workplace action 15

    Drink–driving policies and countermeasures 18

    Availability of alcohol 20

    Marketing of alcoholic beverages 22

    Pricing policies 24

    Reducing the negative consequences of drinking and
alcohol intoxication 26

    Reducing the public health impact of illicit alcohol and
informally produced alcohol 28

    Monitoring and surveillance 30

Role of the WHO Regional Office for Europe 33

Annexes 37

Annex 1. WHO Regional Committee for Europe resolution EUR/RC61/R4 39

Annex 2. Indicators 43

Annex 3. Checklist for policy response 73

Foreword

The European Region of WHO has the unenviable position of being the region of the world with the highest levels of alcohol consumption and alcohol-related harm. This is a challenge. Relatively simple and inexpensive action can, however, bring rapid and considerable gains in population health and well-being, enhanced employment and productivity, increased health and social welfare savings, greater health and economic equality, and greater social cohesion and inclusion. A public health response is, therefore, feasible and effective.

With its first European alcohol action plan in 1992, the European Region has been at the forefront in providing leadership to reduce the harm done by alcohol. Spurred on by the momentum for action brought on by the 2010 global strategy to reduce the harmful use of alcohol, the Region can maintain this world leadership role through the launch of a re-invigorated European action plan to reduce the harmful use of alcohol 2012–2020.

The importance of the harmful use of alcohol as a public health priority, with action integral to successful promotion of well-being and healthy lifestyles and reduction of the burden of noncommunicable disease, as well as some communicable diseases, should never be underestimated. Even though only half the world's population drinks alcohol, it is the third leading cause of ill health and premature death globally, after low birth weight and unsafe sex, and greater than tobacco. Alcohol is teratogenic, affecting the developing fetus; neurotoxic, affecting brain development; intoxicating, causing a wide range of intentional and unintentional injuries; carcinogenic, causing a wide range of cancers; an immunosuppressant, increasing the risk of communicable diseases, and a cause of a range of cardiovascular diseases. Alcohol harms people other than the drinker, whether through violence, traffic accidents, domestic violence in the family, or simply using up government resources. The greater the exposure to heavy drinking, the greater the impact on quality of life. Economic efficiency is impaired through diminished productivity due to alcohol. The real risk of dying from an alcohol-related condition increases with the amount of alcohol consumed over a lifetime, with heavy drinking occasions (when most alcohol is drunk) being particularly risky.

The action plan was endorsed by 53 European Member States at the Regional Committee for Europe in September 2011 in Baku, Azerbaijan. It includes a wide range of policies and programmes that are relatively easy and cheap to implement, can reduce the harmful use of alcohol, promote health and well-being, improve productivity, and enhance human, health and social capital across the life course from birth to old age. This action plan proposes a range of options for the 10 action areas of the global strategy to reduce the harmful use of alcohol that all European Member States can engage in.

With leadership and commitment, all Member States can strengthen their actions on alcohol and subsequently gain from the resulting health and economic rewards.

Zsuzsanna Jakab
WHO Regional Director for Europe

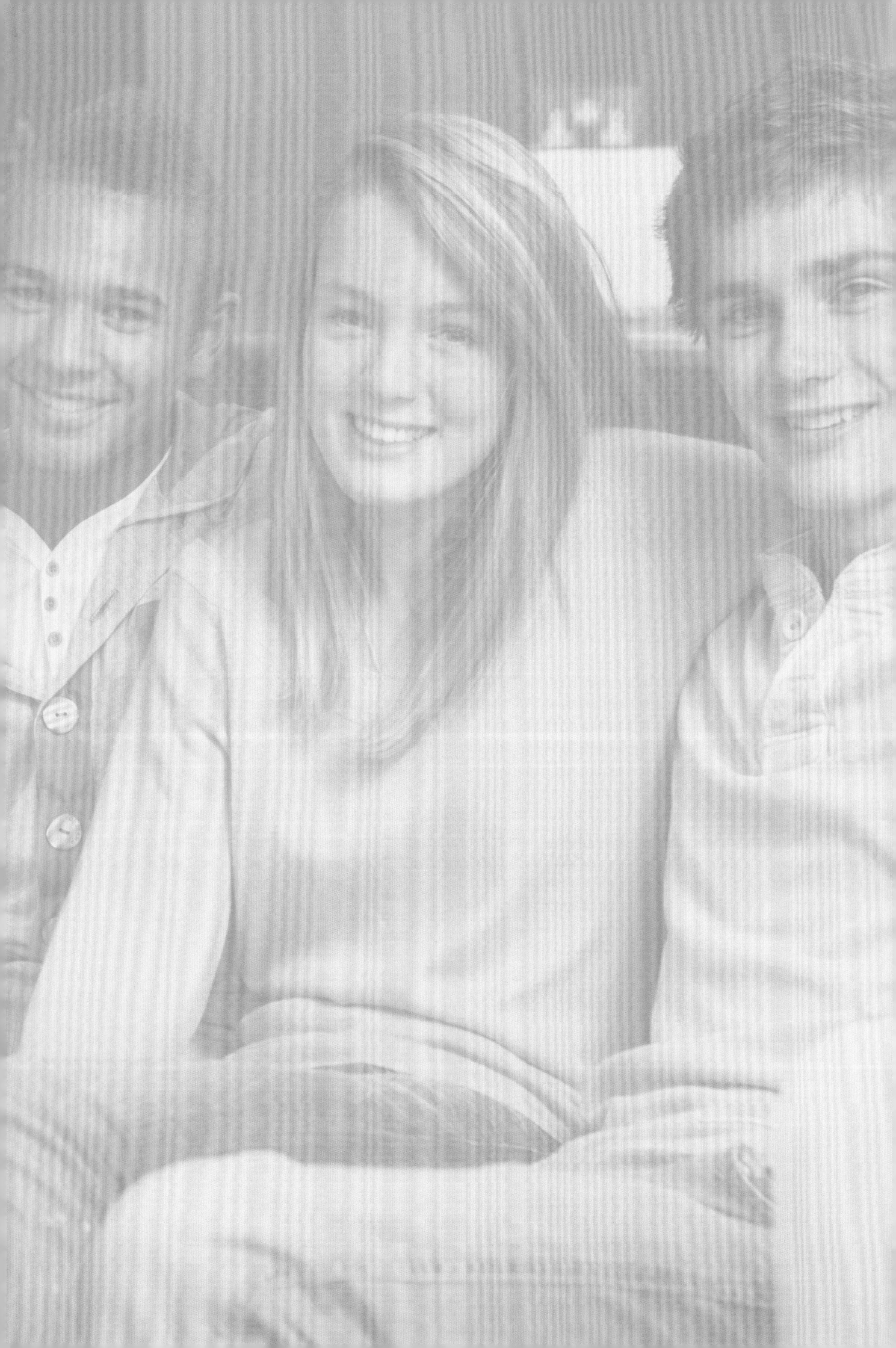

The European action plan to reduce the harmful use of alcohol 2012–2020

The need for strengthened action in Europe

Countries that take stronger action on alcohol will reap considerable gains in terms of better population health and well-being, enhanced employment and productivity, increased health and social welfare savings, greater health and economic equality, and greater social cohesion and inclusion.

Impact of the harmful use of alcohol on health and well-being

Alcohol is one of the world's top three priority public health areas. The evidence available to support this statement is large, diverse and persuasive. Even though only half the world's population drinks alcohol, it is the world's third leading cause of ill health and premature death, after low birth weight and unsafe sex (for which alcohol is a risk factor), and greater than tobacco. Alcohol impacts on both noncommunicable and communicable diseases. A reinvigorated European action plan is all the more important given that WHO's European Region remains the area of the world with the highest levels of alcohol consumption and alcohol-related harm. In the Region, 40% of poor health and premature deaths are caused by three avoidable risk factors: smoking, alcohol and traffic accidents (which are in turn frequently caused by alcohol). Alcohol-related cardiovascular and injury mortalities are a major cause of health inequalities between Member States.

Most alcohol is drunk in heavy drinking occasions, which worsen all risks. In particular, heavy drinking occasions are a cause of all types of intentional and unintentional injuries, and of ischaemic heart disease and sudden death. Alcohol harms people other than the drinker, whether through violence on the street, domestic violence in the family, or simply using up government resources, notably through the costs of providing health care and dealing with crime and

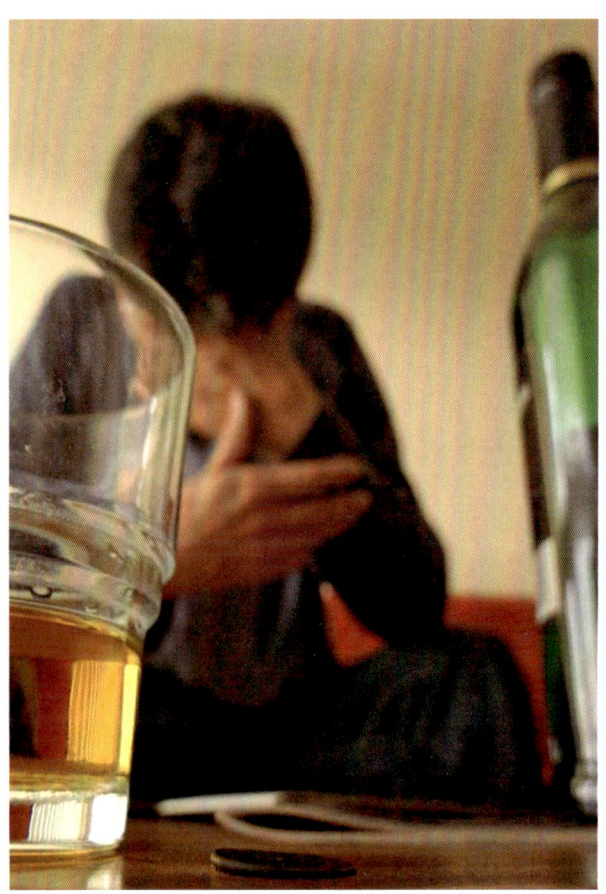

disorder. Up to three in ten people may have someone in their life who is a heavy drinker.

Including the harm done by alcohol from someone else's drinking is likely to double the social costs of alcohol. The external impact and costs of the harmful use of alcohol are thus considerably greater than those associated with smoking (environmental tobacco smoke) and far greater than those of illicit drugs. Who you are and where you live are important. Socially disadvantaged people and people who live in socially disadvantaged areas experience more harm from alcohol than the better-off. Increased spending on social welfare policies can mitigate the impact of economic recession and unemployment on increased alcohol-related deaths.

Economic efficiency is impaired through diminished productivity due to alcohol. It used to be thought that individuals with low to moderate levels of alcohol consumption had higher earnings than abstainers. However, a fuller analysis of these results finds that this is an artefact and that there is no level of alcohol consumption that has a positive impact on wages. Rather, it seems that low to moderate alcohol consumption is a proxy for a range of personality traits that have a positive influence on human capital.

The real absolute risk of dying from an adverse alcohol-related condition increases with the total amount of alcohol consumed over a lifetime. For many conditions, including alcohol-related cancers, the risk is increased at even low levels of consumption. Studies have shown that middle-aged and older light to moderate drinkers are less likely to die from ischaemic events (coronary heart disease, ischaemic stroke and type 2 diabetes) than abstainers. This effect is found to be equal for people who just drink beer or who just drink wine. However, more and more it is understood that a large part of this effect is due to confounders, with low to moderate alcohol use being a proxy for better health and social capital. Thus, it seems that the real protective effect is lower and occurs at a lower dose of alcohol than previously thought. In any case, there is no protective effect for younger people, where any dose of alcohol increases the risk of ischaemic events. And in older people, a greater reduction in death from ischaemic heart disease could be obtained by being physically active and eating a healthier diet than by drinking a low dose of alcohol.

Alcohol can diminish individual health and human capital across the lifespan from the embryo to old age. In absolute terms, it is mostly the middle-aged (and men in particular) who die from alcohol. However, taking into account a life-course view, exposure to alcohol during pregnancy can impair the brain development of the fetus and is associated with intellectual deficits that become apparent later in childhood. The adolescent brain is particularly susceptible to alcohol and the longer the onset

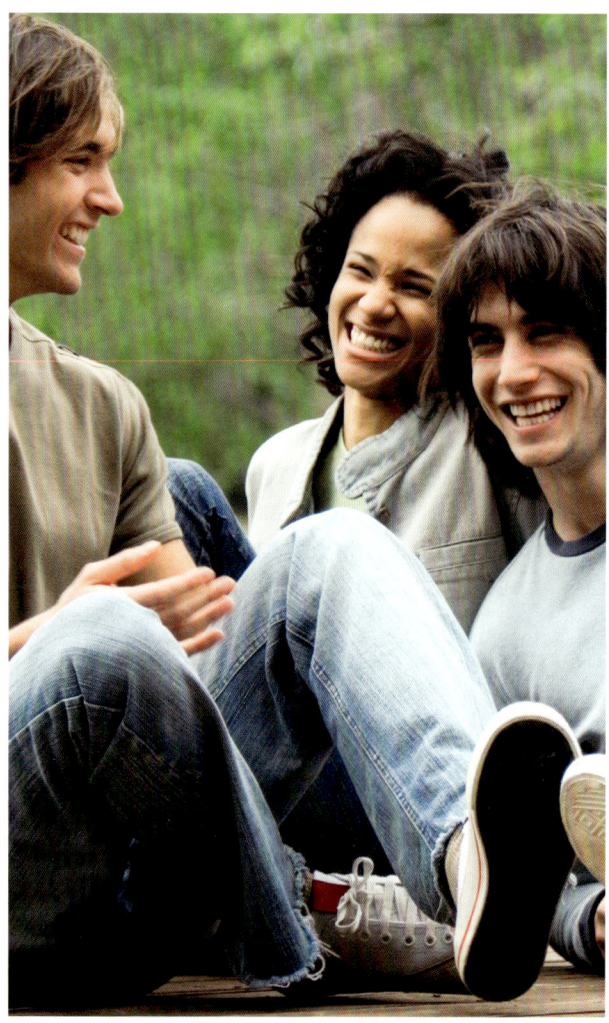

of consumption is delayed, the less likely it is that problems and alcohol dependence will emerge in adult life. Alcohol is also an intoxicant affecting a wide range of structures and processes in the central nervous system which, interacting with personality characteristics, associated behaviour and sociocultural expectations, are causal factors for intentional and unintentional injuries, harm to people other than the drinker and drink–driving fatalities. In the workplace, harmful alcohol use and heavy episodic drinking increase the risk of problems such as absenteeism, low productivity and inappropriate behaviour, and can also increase the risk of alcohol use disorders and alcohol dependence.

Building on a momentum of action

The important thing about alcohol is that effective measures and policies exist to reduce harms and achieve gains, with almost immediate effect. Europe has been at the forefront of action to reduce the harm done by alcohol. The European Region of WHO was the first region to approve an alcohol action plan, in 1992 and again in 2000. In 2001, a ministerial conference on alcohol and young people was organized in Stockholm, Sweden, with the adoption of a declaration on young people and alcohol. In 2005, at the fifty-fifth session of the WHO Regional Committee for Europe, the action plan was succeeded by the framework for alcohol policy, maintaining and reinforcing the core principles and measures in the action plan.

In 2006, the European Commission launched its Communication on an EU strategy to support Member States in reducing alcohol-related harm, with a focus on protecting young people, children and the unborn child; reducing injuries and death from alcohol-related road accidents; preventing alcohol-related harm among adults and reducing the negative impact on the workplace; informing, educating and raising awareness about the impact of harmful and hazardous alcohol consumption and about appropriate consumption patterns; and developing and maintaining a common evidence base at EU level.

By adopting resolution WHA63.13 in 2010, the Sixty-third World Health Assembly endorsed the global strategy to reduce the harmful use of alcohol, urged Member States to adopt and implement the global strategy as appropriate, and requested the Director-General to give sufficiently high organizational priority, and to assure adequate financial and human resources at all levels, to prevention and reduction of the harmful use of alcohol and implementation of the global strategy; to collaborate with and provide support to Member States, as appropriate, in implementing the global strategy to reduce the harmful use of alcohol and strengthening national responses to public health problems caused by the harmful use of alcohol; and to monitor progress in implementing the global strategy. It is thus timely to build on this momentum and reinvigorate regional action with a new European action plan to reduce the harmful use of alcohol 2012–2020.

The European action plan is closely linked to the interventions in the action plan for implementation of the European Strategy for the Prevention and Control of Noncommunicable Diseases (2012–2016) but is more detailed in its targets and action. The action plan is also closely linked to the new European health policy, Health 2020, where noncommunicable diseases and the risk factors behind them are a priority for WHO during 2012–2020.

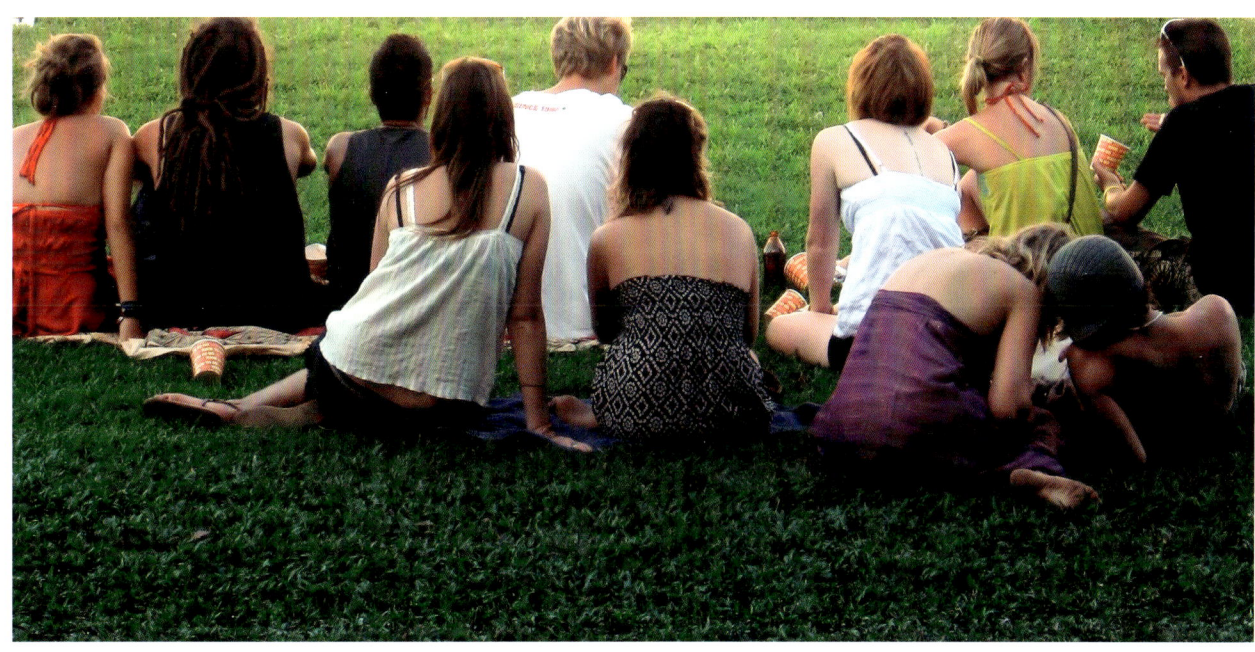

Policy response in Europe

Policy response to date

While there is extensive activity to reduce the harmful use of alcohol at the level of Member States, there is still considerable room for improvement. *The European status report on alcohol and health,*[1] which can act as a baseline for this action plan, notes that four out of ten countries did not have a written national alcohol policy in 2009, and only six out of ten countries produced regular monitoring reports, but on a diffuse range of non-standardized indicators. Of the 45 Member States which responded to the survey, 27 have adopted a national alcohol policy and two thirds of them have done this since 2005 when the latest WHO Regional Committee for Europe resolution on alcohol (EUR/RC55/R1) was adopted.

Most countries were implementing national awareness activities, and countries had generally taken effective action on drink–driving, with only a small number of countries arguably in need of reducing their legal maximum blood alcohol levels for driving. When it came to the more cost–effective policy options, the picture was less encouraging, with a significant number of countries imposing no restrictions on alcohol advertising, and enforcement generally considered to be in need of improvement. Overall, restrictions on availability remained poor, and in one third of countries adolescents under the age of 18 years could freely purchase alcohol. Generally, alcohol taxes represented a low proportion of the retail price and, relative to the consumer price index, alcohol prices were at the same level or had decreased in over half the countries during the previous five years.

Standing back, it can be said that alcohol policies still do not reflect the gravity of the health, social and economic harm resulting from the harmful use of alcohol; they fail to be properly integrated within overall health, social and development policies; and they fail to provide adequate capacity to ensure policy coherence and "joined-up" action between different

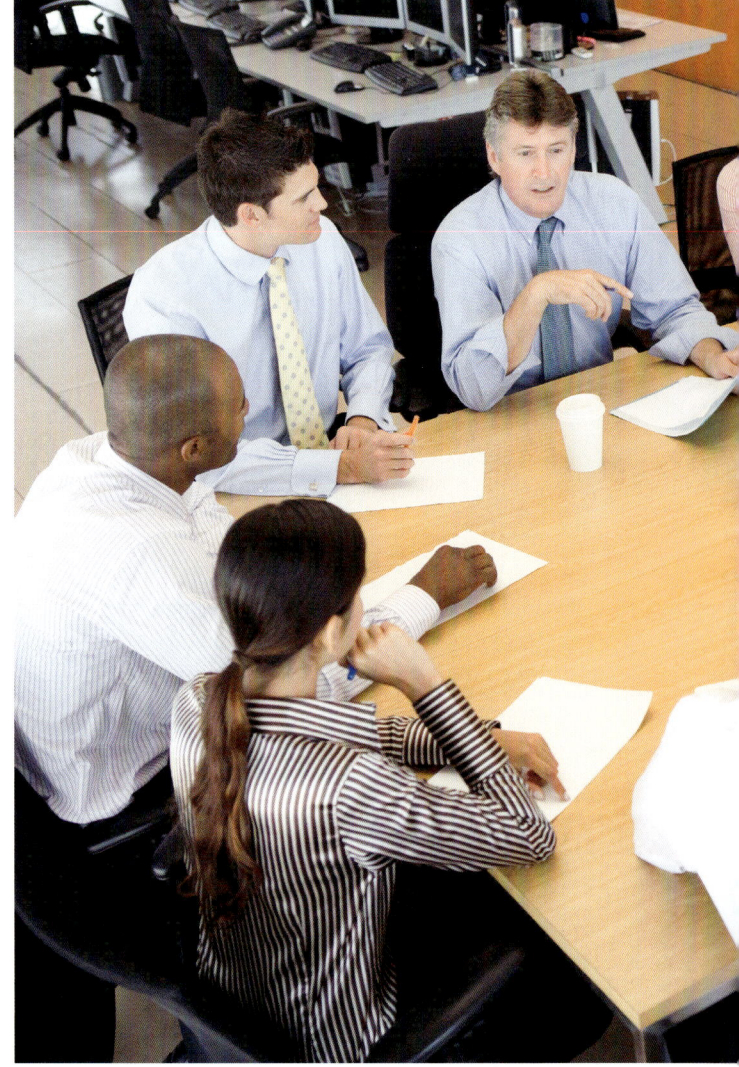

government departments and sectors and at all levels of jurisdiction.

Policy for the future

There is no doubt that there is a rapidly building momentum for countries, individually and collectively, to take more effective action to reduce the harmful use of alcohol, spurred on by the global strategy launched in 2010. Those countries that are most active in implementing evidence-based and cost–effective

---

[1] *European status report on alcohol and health 2010.* Copenhagen, WHO Regional Office for Europe, 2010 (http://www.euro.who.int/__data/assets/pdf_file/0004/128065/e94533.pdf, accessed 16 June 2011).

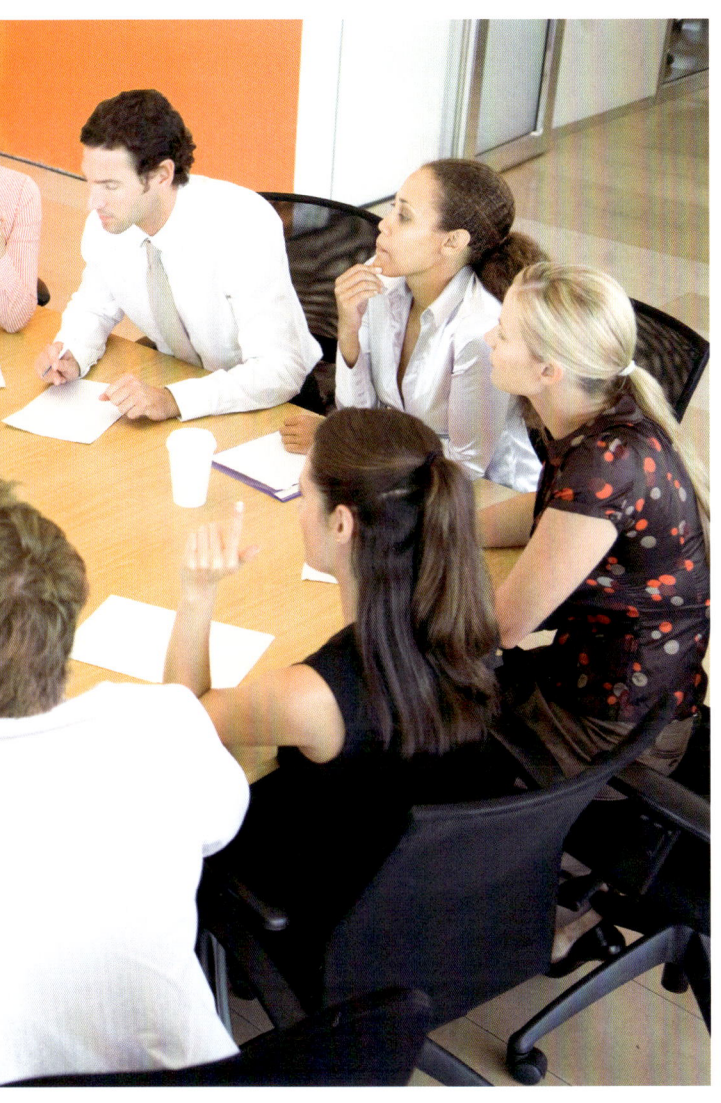

alcohol policies and programmes will profit from substantial gains in health and well-being, productivity and social development. Given that many alcohol policy issues readily cross European borders, coherent action across countries will bring added value. Further, international frameworks should enable, rather than hinder, individual countries to be bold and innovative in taking evidence-based approaches to reducing the harmful use of alcohol. Supporting the needs of the 53 Member States in the European Region, WHO's public health mandate affords the opportunity to propose a wide range of options for Member State action to reduce the harmful use of alcohol.

Effective alcohol policy over the coming years will have a number of attributes, reflecting the two-way processes and interactions between effective alcohol policy, social development and social capital. In other words, it is not possible to have effective social development leading to improved human, health and social capital without effective alcohol policy, and it is not possible to reduce alcohol-related harm without improved human, health and social capital. Further, adequate human, health and social capital are prerequisites for the societal resilience necessary to mitigate future global stressors that will impinge on the health of the European Region as a consequence of, for example, climate change.[2]

Effective future alcohol policy will be that which ensures:

- integration of alcohol polices into broad economic and welfare policies, contributing to the effective development of societies' social, health and economic well-being;
- coherence and "joined-up" action between different government departments and sectors, identifying and implementing the necessary incentives that give gains to individual sectors and society as a whole;
- coherence and involvement of public and private actors alike, also identifying and implementing the incentives that benefit relevant public and private actors;
- integration of alcohol policy measures into all actions that promote well-being and healthy lifestyles and that reduce the burden of noncommunicable and communicable diseases;
- the capacity and opportunity for municipalities, local communities and civil society to implement effective alcohol policies and programmes that are aligned across all levels of society;

---

[2] *Protecting health in an environment challenged by climate change: European Regional Framework for Action.* Copenhagen, WHO Regional Office for Europe, 2010 (document EUR/55934/6 Rev.1, http://www.euro.who.int/__data/assets/pdf_file/0005/95882/Parma_EH_Conf_edoc06rev1.pdf, accessed 16 June 2011).

- the provision of incentives, as well as disincentives, for individuals and families to make more healthful choices when it comes to the use of alcohol;
- tackling the demand side and responding to the role that alcohol plays alongside other factors in people's lives; and
- the recognition that everyone has a role to play whether individuals, communities, local health care and social care organizations, nongovernmental organizations (NGOs), the alcohol industry and government.

Objectives

Building on previous European alcohol action plans, the five main objectives of the present action plan are aligned with those of the global strategy to:

- raise awareness of the magnitude and nature of the health, social and economic burdens of the harmful use of alcohol, and to foster increased government commitment to addressing those burdens;
- strengthen and disseminate the knowledge base on the size and determinants of alcohol-related harm and on effective interventions to reduce and prevent that harm;
- increase technical support to, and enhance the capacity of, Member States for reducing the harm done by alcohol, and managing and treating alcohol use disorders and associated health conditions;
- strengthen partnerships and improve coordination among stakeholders and increase mobilization of resources required for concerted action to reduce the harmful use of alcohol; and
- improve systems for monitoring and surveillance at subnational, national and European levels, and ensure more effective dissemination and application of information for advocacy, policy development and evaluation.

Action and outcomes

All European countries have some form of alcohol regulation or plan. However, the comprehensiveness of those regulations or plans varies, as does the experience of each country, area and municipality in implementing them. No matter how comprehensive or strict its alcohol action plan may be, every country is likely to benefit from reviewing, adjusting and strengthening it.

A national alcohol action plan or strategy is needed to establish priorities and guide action. National health goals can set priorities, express commitment to new action and allocate resources. Such goals and priorities should be based on epidemiological evidence, while the choice of strategies and interventions should also be evidence-based. Measures to restrict supply (drink–driving policies and countermeasures, alcohol marketing policies, alcohol taxes, restrictions on outlet density and on days and hours of sale, a minimum purchase age) and to reduce demand (early detection and brief interventions in health care and the workplace, treatment and rehabilitation programmes) are some specific examples of how to reduce alcohol-related harm.

The 10 action points below adhere to the titles and follow the order of the action points included in the WHO global strategy to reduce the harmful use of alcohol. They recommend a portfolio of policy options and measures to be considered for implementation and adjusted as appropriate at the national level, taking into account national circumstances such as religious and cultural contexts and national public health priorities, as well as resources, capacities and capabilities. The main areas are:

- leadership, awareness and commitment;
- health services' response;
- community and workplace action;
- drink–driving policies and countermeasures;
- availability of alcohol;
- marketing of alcoholic beverages;
- pricing policies;
- reducing the negative consequences of drinking and alcohol intoxication;
- reducing the public health impact of illicit alcohol and informally produced alcohol; and
- monitoring and surveillance.

Each action point starts with a headline statement, and includes one or more outcomes and appropriate indicators. A brief background paragraph is followed

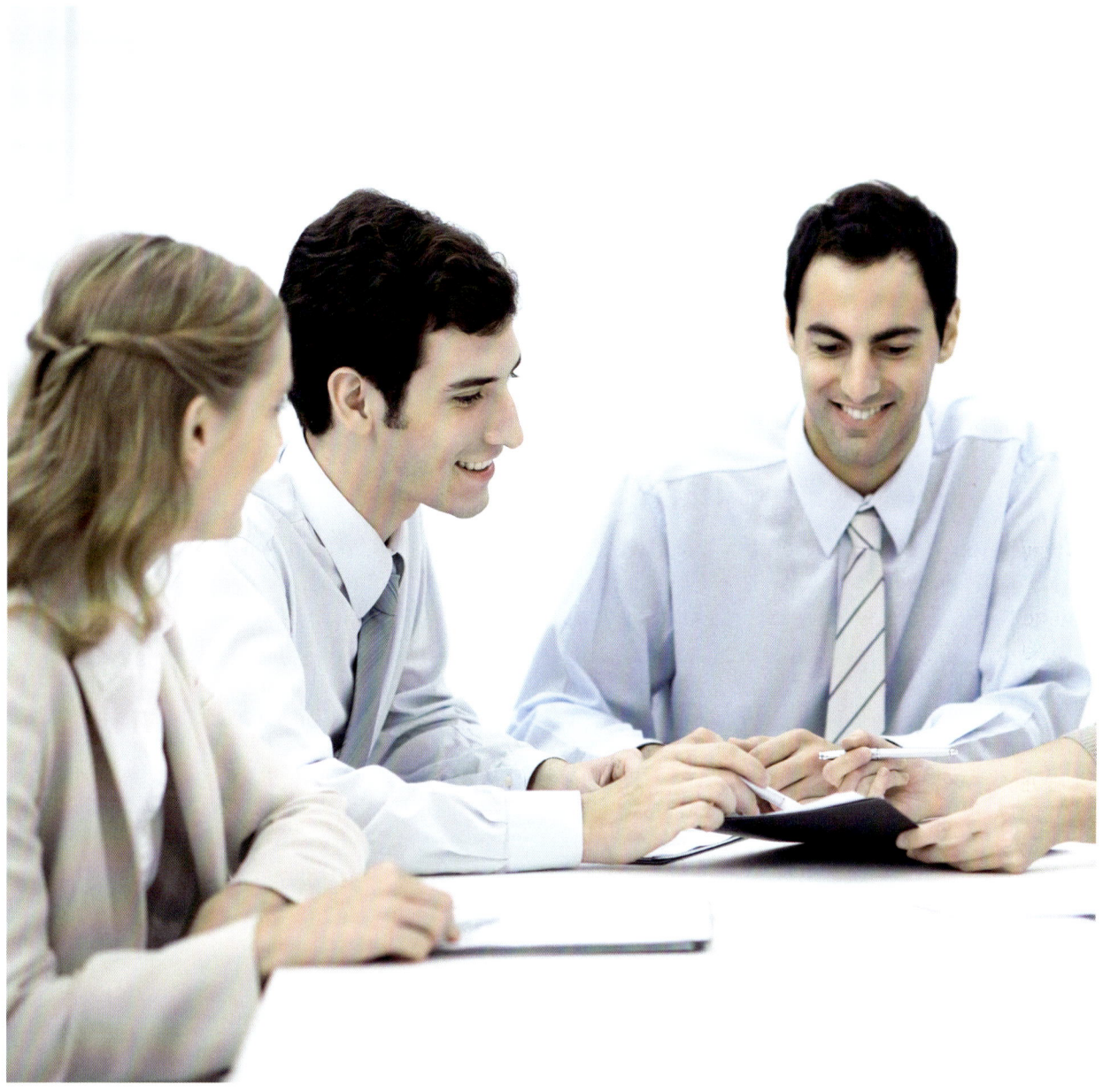

by a discussion of strategies. Finally, a number of options for action are listed. The proposed actions and the evidence behind them are based on two WHO publications from 2009.[3,4]

Each Member State will need to consider the nature of the alcohol-related problems it faces and to determine which of the possible actions listed would prove to be most applicable and effective in its own circumstances. There is no single model that can be applied across the European Region. What matters most is that Member States take the actions most likely to reduce the harm that is caused by alcohol in their countries.

---

[3] *Evidence for the effectiveness and cost–effectiveness of interventions to reduce alcohol-related harm*. Copenhagen, WHO Regional Office for Europe, 2009 (http://www.euro.who.int/__data/assets/pdf_file/0020/43319/E92823.pdf, accessed 16 June 2011).

[4] *Handbook for action to reduce alcohol-related harm*. Copenhagen, WHO Regional Office for Europe, 2009 (http://www.euro.who.int/__data/assets/pdf_file/0012/43320/E92820.pdf, accessed 16 June 2011).

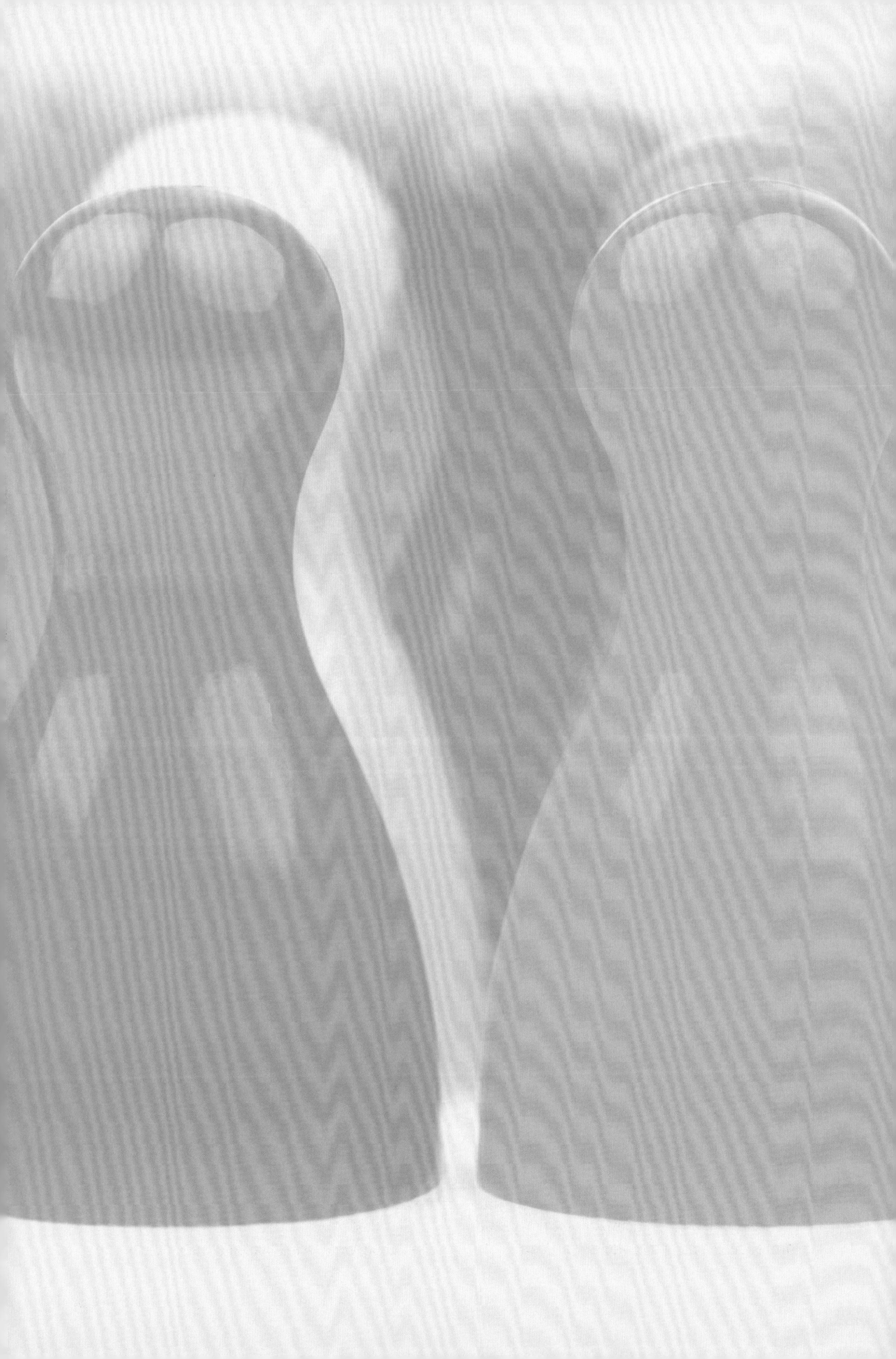

Ten action areas

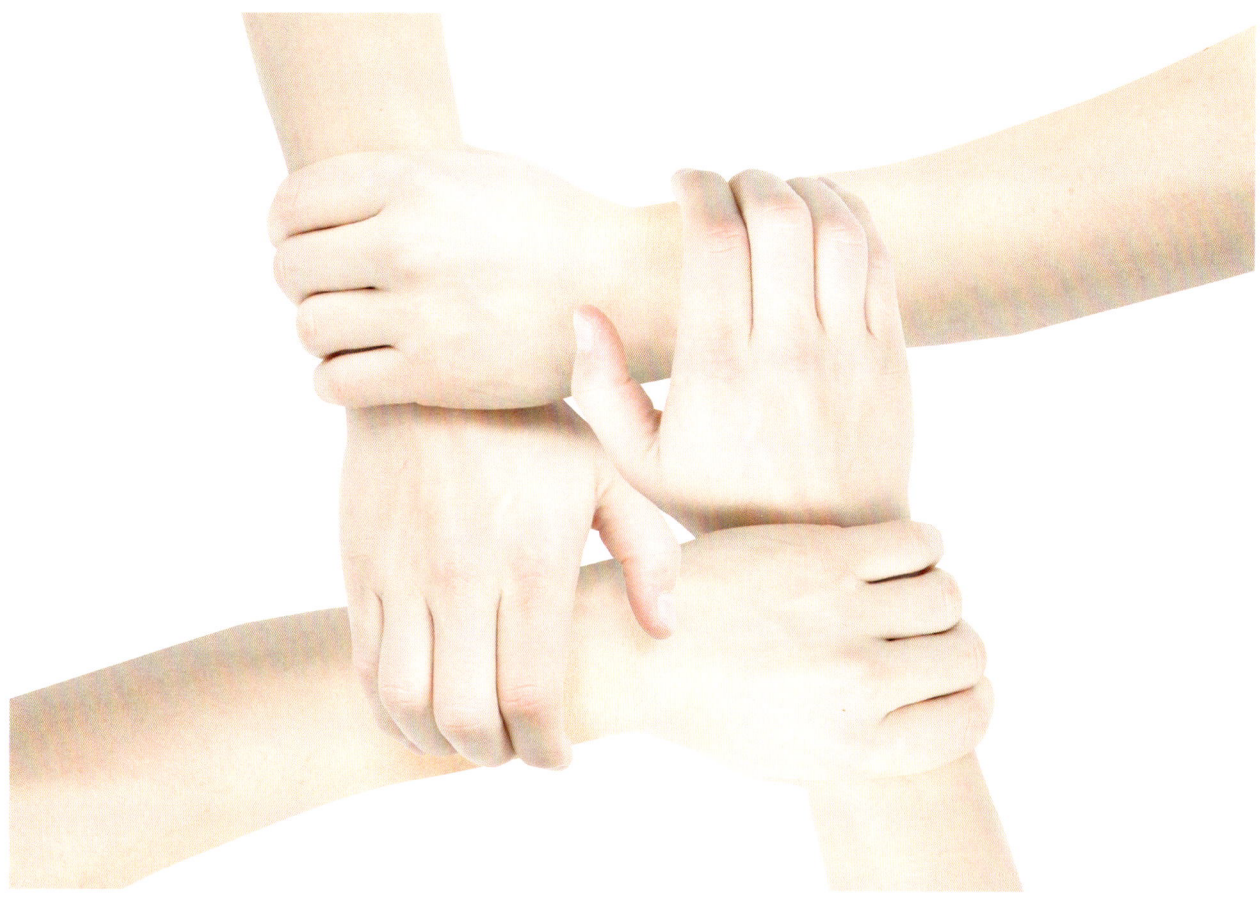

Leadership, awareness and commitment

Headline

The substantial gains that can be made through the implementation of effective alcohol policy can only be achieved through adequate leadership provided by national and local government to ensure the full awareness and commitment of all sectors and levels of society to reap the gains from sustained and coherent action that reduces the harmful use of alcohol. This is best achieved through comprehensive action plans as "agents" of awareness and through well-informed and supportive societies.

Outcomes

Throughout the duration of this action plan, countries prepare, implement, review and revise at least once an identifiable national action plan or strategy on alcohol. Countries ensure that their populations are progressively informed about the harm that alcohol can do to individuals, families and communities and about the measures that can be taken to reduce that harm.

Indicators

Indicators would include the presence of a publicly accessible national action plan or strategy on alcohol or an alcohol plan included in a national public health plan, and measures of knowledge, attitudes and opinions about alcohol and alcohol policy through barometer surveys and opinion polls of random samples of the population.

Background

For an action plan on reducing alcohol-related harm to be effective, it is necessary to ensure that the requisite infrastructure for policy development, priority-setting, monitoring and surveillance, research and evaluation, workforce development and programme delivery is in place. Despite advances in building core infrastructure for action on alcohol, it can be argued that there continues to be insufficient political will and investment by both the private and the public sectors in many Member States. Ensuring that this infrastructure is sufficiently large and capable remains a challenge.

Many national alcohol strategies and initiatives underscore the need to inform and educate the public. This may express a simple principle that consumers ought to be provided with information and that a population should know about and understand alcohol and its health risks, but it may also reflect the view, contradicted by evidence, that information and education alone can solve alcohol-related problems. In practice, alcohol education rarely goes beyond providing information about the risks to promote the availability of help for alcohol use disorders or to mobilize public support for effective alcohol policies.

Strategies

A national alcohol action plan or strategy is needed to establish priorities and guide action. National health goals can set priorities, express commitment to new action and allocate resources. Such goals and priorities should be based on epidemiological evidence, while the choice of policies and interventions should also be evidence-based. Measurable outcomes make policy objectives more specific, allowing progress to be monitored and often inspiring partners to support policy initiatives. Accountability for the health impact of alcohol actions and programmes rests with all sectors of society, as well as with the government officials who prepare action plans, allocate resources and initiate legislation or non-legal frameworks such as guidelines or voluntary restraints, monitored by co-regulatory frameworks. To enable transparency and accountability, measurable outcomes can be published nationally and, where possible, locally.

The responsibility of the national government for developing and implementing an action plan on alcohol is usually split among several government departments and levels. The departments involved can include those devoted to industry and trade, agriculture, employment, finance and health. The interests and priorities of these different sectors often need to be aligned to produce an agreed alcohol policy, and some sectors may wield disproportionate power. Coordination is needed to ensure that all levels of government and all affected sectors and stakeholders are considered when making decisions on alcohol policy. A coordinating body, such as a national alcohol council, should include senior representatives of ministries, health professionals and other partners.

Public and political support for the content of alcohol action plans is crucial. National politicians have the authority to regulate and influence the environment in which alcohol is marketed. Politicians often have a particular interest in alcohol issues, which can vary according to their official roles as well as their personal views. Contacts with players outside government, such as the alcohol industry or health groups, may shape politicians' views on specific alcohol policies and possibly influence the forming or refining of policy proposals. Responses from civil society and public opinion can impact on alcohol policy reform. In addition to governments, health and medical professionals and institutions supporting public health-oriented alcohol policy include independent, publicly-funded institutions, insurance industry programmes, issue-based NGOs and networks, and professional public health associations.

Information-based public education campaigns about alcohol and responsible drinking behaviour should be proportionate and should concentrate on providing information about the risks of alcohol and the availability of help and treatment to reduce harmful use. Public education programmes should also be used to support alcohol policy measures, particularly when new measures are introduced, such as a reduced blood alcohol limit for driving, an increase in the minimum age for purchasing alcohol or tax increases on alcohol. Web-based information programmes, "audit-testing" and self-help guidance represent new channels of information.

Options for action

Countries need to ensure adequate public health infrastructures for alcohol policy, including political will and a demand for good governance. They must

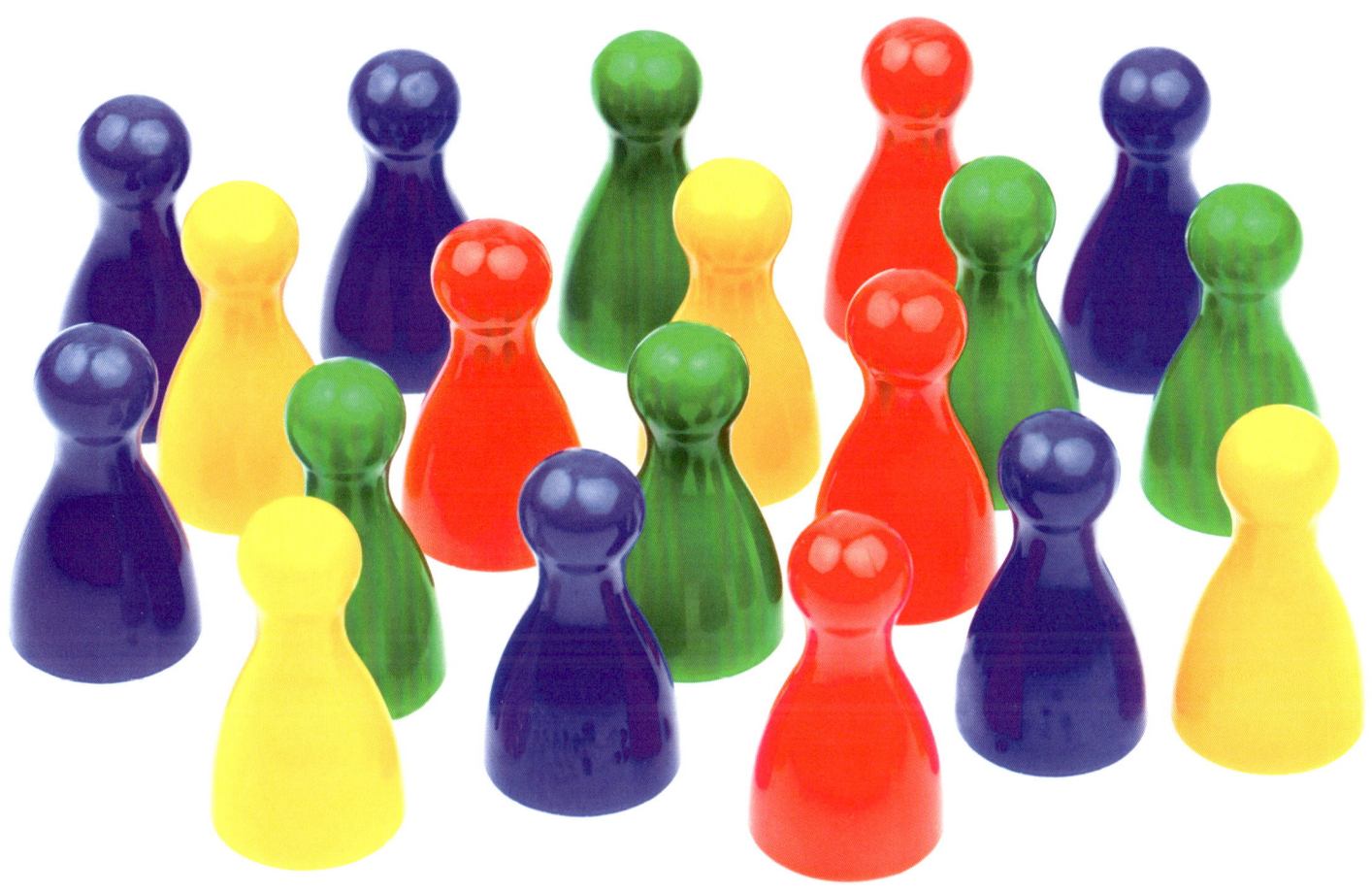

also ensure that adequate resources are allocated to government officials responsible for preventing and managing the harmful use of alcohol, that capacity-building measures are taken in alcohol policy and research, and that knowledge of evidence is introduced into policy and programme practice in all sectors and at all levels. Developed policies need to be comprehensive, minimizing any negative consequences. A lack of transparency and information, poor organization and preparation for the introduction of new policies and laws, a lack of financing, the presence of corruption and public distrust of authority are all impediments to the acceptance, implementation and enforcement of effective policy. As a minimum, countries would be expected to have an identifiable national action plan or strategy on alcohol, including measurable health and policy outcomes; a coordinating body or mechanism to promote policy coherence and joined-up action across relevant government departments and sectors, and an adequately resourced nongovernmental sector, free of potential conflict of interest with the public health interest, to give voice to civil society.

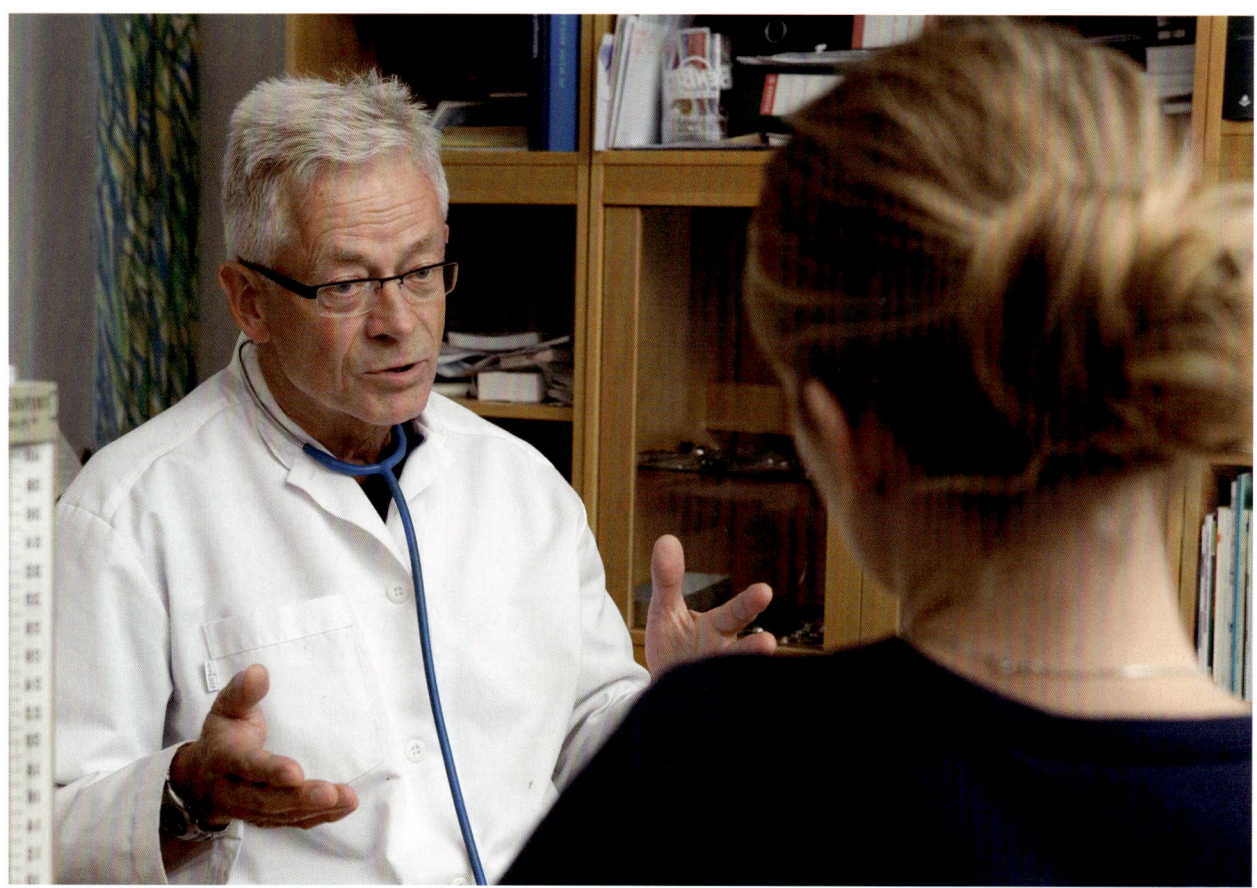

Health services' response

Headline

The health sector and, through its support, the social welfare, education and workplace sectors have real opportunities to reap both health gains and financial savings through the widespread implementation of brief advice programmes that have been shown to reduce ill health and premature death subsequent to hazardous and harmful alcohol consumption,[5] and the implementation of evidence-based treatment programmes for alcohol use disorders. Emphasis should also be placed on helping to reduce alcohol consumption during pregnancy, and on protecting family members other than the drinker and children from the consequences of alcohol dependence and alcohol-related harm. This requires leadership from governments and health insurance companies to provide the incentives for providers from different settings to take the required action.

Outcome

Throughout the duration of this action plan, countries should progressively reduce the gap between the number of people who would benefit from alcohol consumption advice to reduce or prevent harm, engagement in social rehabilitation programmes or treatment for alcohol use disorder and the number who actually receive such advice or treatment.

Indicator

Indicators would include the proportion of the adult population with hazardous and harmful alcohol consumption, and the proportion of the population with hazardous and harmful alcohol consumption who have received therapy and advice from a primary care provider to reduce their alcohol intake.

---

[5] Considered as consumption greater than 40 g alcohol per day for a man and 30 g alcohol per day for a woman.

Background

Alcohol use disorders, including harmful alcohol use and alcohol dependence, are officially classified in the list of mental and behavioural disorders in the International Statistical Classification of Diseases and Related Health Problems, 10th revision (ICD-10). In general, the prevalence of alcohol use disorders is quite high, with, in most countries, perhaps one in six adults drinking at least 40 g alcohol per day for a man and 30 g for a woman, and some 1 in 16 adults suffering from alcohol dependence in any given year. In almost every country studied, there is a considerable gap between the number of people who would benefit from alcohol consumption advice, engagement in social rehabilitation programmes or treatment and the number of them who actually receive such advice or treatment. It has been estimated that only 1 in 20 of those with hazardous or harmful alcohol use are actually identified and offered brief advice by a primary care provider; similarly, less than 1 in 20 with a diagnosis of alcohol dependence have actually seen a specialist for treatment.

Strategies

Evidence strongly supports the benefits of widespread implementation of early identification and brief advice programmes for individuals with hazardous and harmful alcohol consumption in primary care, social welfare settings and accident and emergency departments, and of offering programmes in the workplace and educational environments. Governments can support identification and brief advice programmes and referral to specialist services by ensuring that clinical guidelines for such interventions are widely available; that primary care providers receive the training, clinical materials and advice they need to set up such programmes; and that they are adequately reimbursed for the interventions, either as part of quality improvement initiatives or with fee-for-service payments. Primary care providers find it easier to undertake this intervention when they are supported by specialist services to which they can refer difficult-to-manage drinkers. In the management of alcohol use disorders, the transition from primary to specialist care should ideally be seamless. Specialist

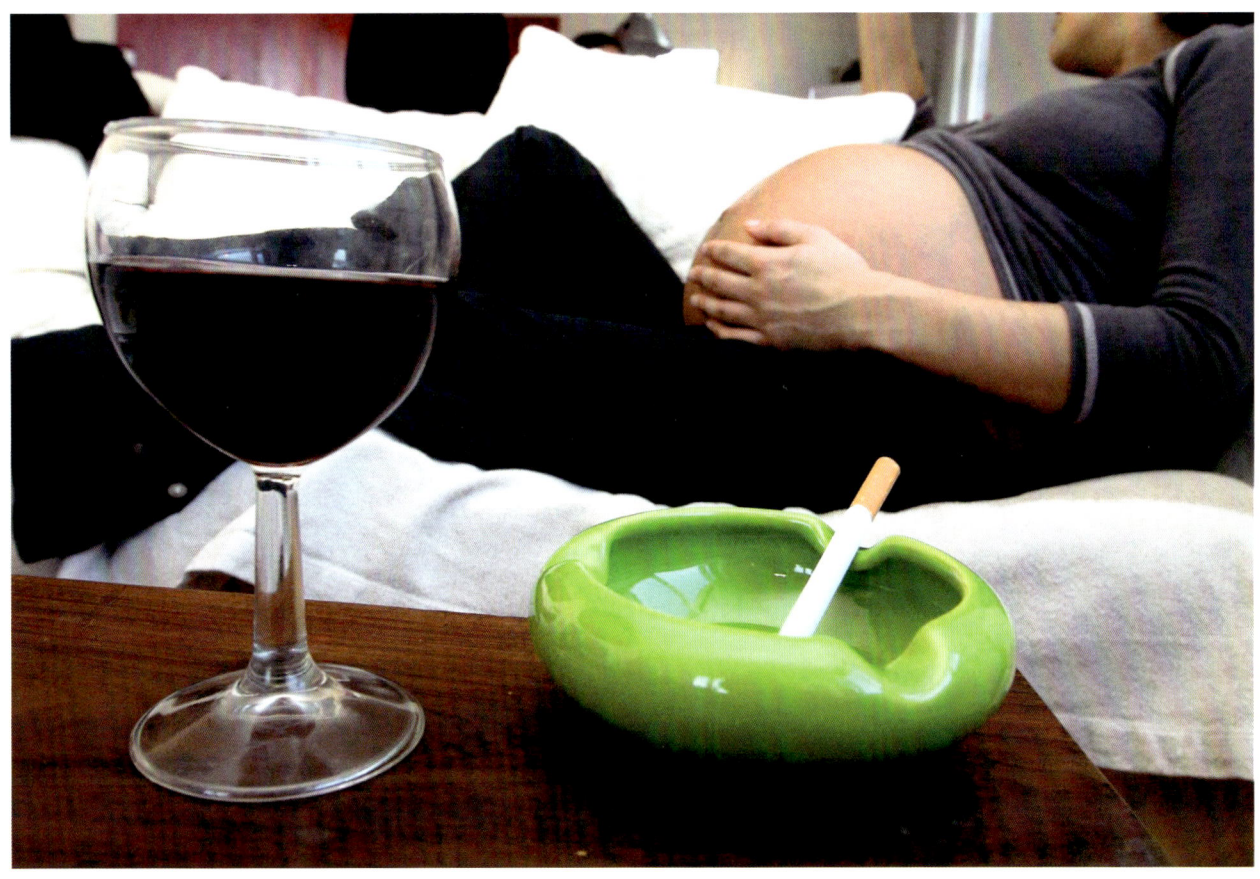

services for managing alcohol withdrawal and treating alcohol use disorders using evidence-based behavioural and pharmacological treatments should be offered to those who have been assessed as likely to benefit. The trend has been to move away from lengthy inpatient treatment towards outpatient and community-based treatment. Compulsory treatment is no longer recommended, except in the case of court-mandated treatment for recidivist drink–drivers, which some evidence has shown can be effective. Midwifery and obstetric services should ensure that all pregnant women are offered information and, if appropriate, advice about drinking during pregnancy, and social welfare services should implement support to help protect family members other than the drinker and children from the harmful consequences of alcohol dependence and alcohol use disorders.

Options for action

All the evidence suggests that the majority of hazardous and harmful drinkers are not receiving advice from primary care providers as a matter of course, and that many people with alcohol use disorders who would benefit from treatment are not currently receiving it. Leaving the situation unchanged might be viewed as costing nothing, but that is a false assumption. Investments in early identification and brief advice programmes not only improve health and save lives, but also save health systems money. Two levels of action can be taken.

- Set a target of offering early identification and brief advice programmes to 30% of the population at risk of hazardous or harmful alcohol consumption. This target could be achieved by putting into place appropriate systems, including provider training, so that every patient who registers with a new primary care provider, receives a health check, consults a provider about particular disease categories (such as hypertension or tuberculosis) or goes to particular types of clinics is offered these interventions. Web-based information and self-help guidance could also be considered.
- Set a target of offering early identification and brief advice programmes to 60% of the population at risk. This more ambitious target would require that every patient who receives primary care services would be offered these interventions, irrespective of the reason for the consultation. It would also necessitate a greater investment in training and supporting primary care providers.

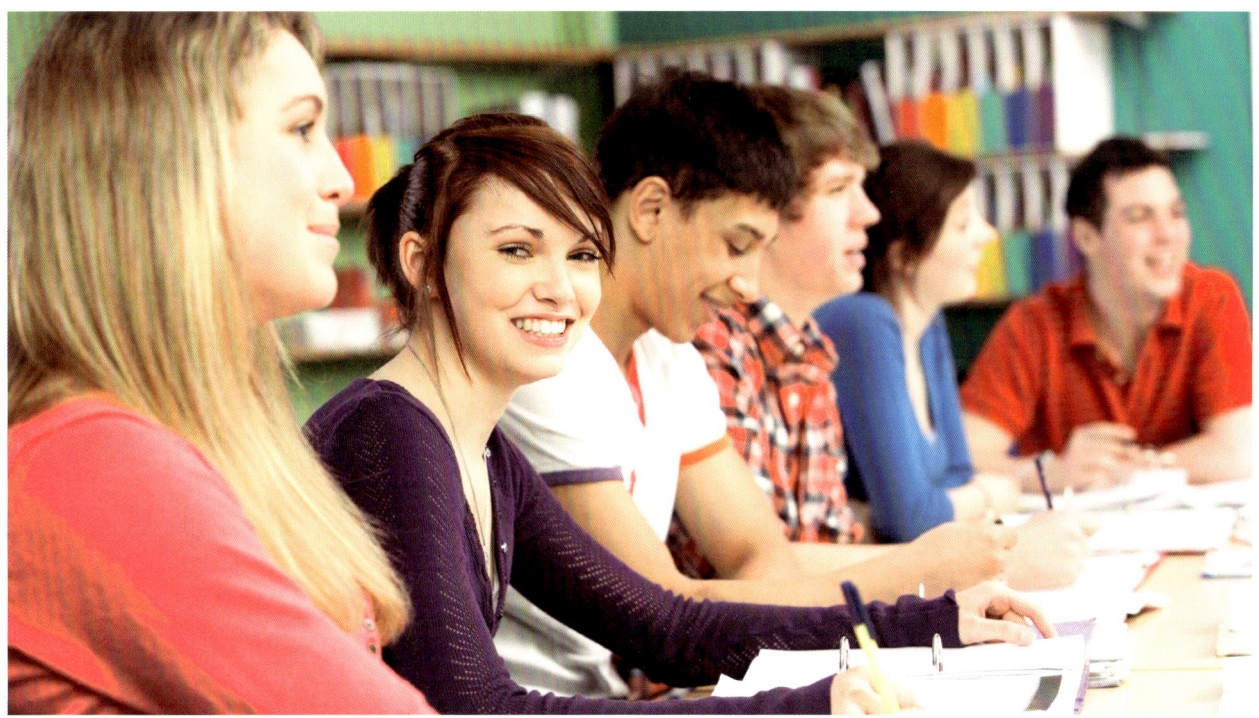

Community and workplace action

Headline

Action at the local level, in communities, workplaces and educational settings, when delivered in a coordinated and aligned manner, can reduce the harmful use of alcohol by changing collective rather than individual behaviour. Public education campaigns and information about health risks given on alcoholic beverage labels can be used to support local action and alcohol policy measures. To be fully effective, local and collective action requires partnership and capacity-building across different sectors and sustained leadership at different levels of society.

Outcomes

Throughout the duration of this action plan, countries should, where appropriate, endeavour progressively to increase the number of schools implementing health-promoting action that includes action on alcohol; the number of municipalities with local action plans on alcohol; and the number of workplaces and employing bodies that implement "alcohol in the workplace" policies and programmes.

Indicators

Indicators would include the proportion of schools, municipalities, and workplaces implementing policies and programmes on alcohol that include specified criteria.

Background

Enacting alcohol policy at the community level has the advantage that alcohol problems have immediate local consequences to which a community must respond directly, such as dealing with injuries and deaths from road traffic accidents, providing hospital and emergency medical services and providing interventions for the harmful use of alcohol and alcohol dependence. It is, therefore, important that municipalities have an alcohol action plan that comprises policies on alcohol in schools and workplaces, a focus on availability through licence control with restaurants and bars, etc. The municipality must also qualify the professionals in the social sector, kindergartens and schools so that they focus on early detection of alcohol problems and referral to brief interventions or alcohol treatment. Communities vary considerably with respect to alcohol problems. An urban setting can be a risk factor for harmful levels and patterns of alcohol use, particularly when it is an area of low social capital, or when it develops a night-time economy and generates high levels of drinking-related nuisance and harassment.

In the workplace, harmful alcohol use and heavy episodic drinking increase the risks for absenteeism, presenteeism (reduced performance at work), arriving at work late, leaving work early, accidents, turnover due to premature death, low productivity, inappropriate behaviour, theft and other crimes that can require disciplinary action, poor co-worker relations and low company morale. Conversely, structural factors at the workplace, including high stress and low satisfaction, can increase the risk of alcohol use disorders and alcohol dependence.

Strategies

Alcohol education should be considered as part of a wider policy approach. It should start at childhood with parenting support and continue in schools as part of the holistic approach of the health-promoting school. Given its limitations, it should be based on educational practices that have proven effective, such as targeting a relevant period in young people's development, talking to young people from the target group during that development phase, testing the intervention with teachers as well as members of the target group, ensuring the programme is interactive and based on skills development, setting behaviour change goals that are relevant for all participants, returning to conduct booster sessions in subsequent years, incorporating information that is of immediate practical use to young people, conducting appropriate teacher training for delivering the material interactively, and making any programme that proves to be effective widely available and marketing it to increase exposure. Family-based programmes could also be considered, because alcohol problems in a family are a problem not only for the drinker but also for the health and well-being of the partner and especially for the development of the children. As part of community-based prevention programmes, it is relevant to qualify those who take care of children (including teachers) in carrying out early interventions among parents with alcohol problems and referral to brief intervention or treatment. This approach will also provide support to partners and children.

Workplace efforts that can reduce alcohol-related harm include policies promoting alcohol-free workplaces, a managerial style that reduces job stress and increases job rewards, and optional workplace interventions that are available on request, such as psychosocial skills training, brief advice and alcohol information programmes.

Community-based prevention programmes can be effective in reducing drink–driving, alcohol-related traffic fatalities and assault injuries. Community mobilization has also been used to raise awareness of problems associated with drinking on licensed premises (such as noise and aggressive behaviour), to develop specific solutions to them and to get establishment owners to acknowledge their community responsibility for addressing them. Evaluation of community mobilization efforts and documentation of grassroots projects suggest that community mobilization can reduce aggression and other problems related to drinking on licensed premises. The main characteristic of effective community programmes is that they implement and mobilize support for interventions known to be effective, such as drink–driving laws or stricter enforcement of restrictions on alcohol sales to minors and intoxicated people.

Options for action

Failure to redirect and coordinate alcohol education initiatives risks continued inappropriate and inefficient use of scarce resources, for instance by using poorly designed and ineffective programmes. Likewise, failing to invest further in community programmes, an opportunity to mobilize public support for new alcohol policy efforts may be lost. In addition, it is likely that many existing community and workplace programmes have not been designed or implemented optimally, or have not been evaluated. A wide range of actions are possible.

Steps should be taken to redesign and reinvest in school-based education and public information

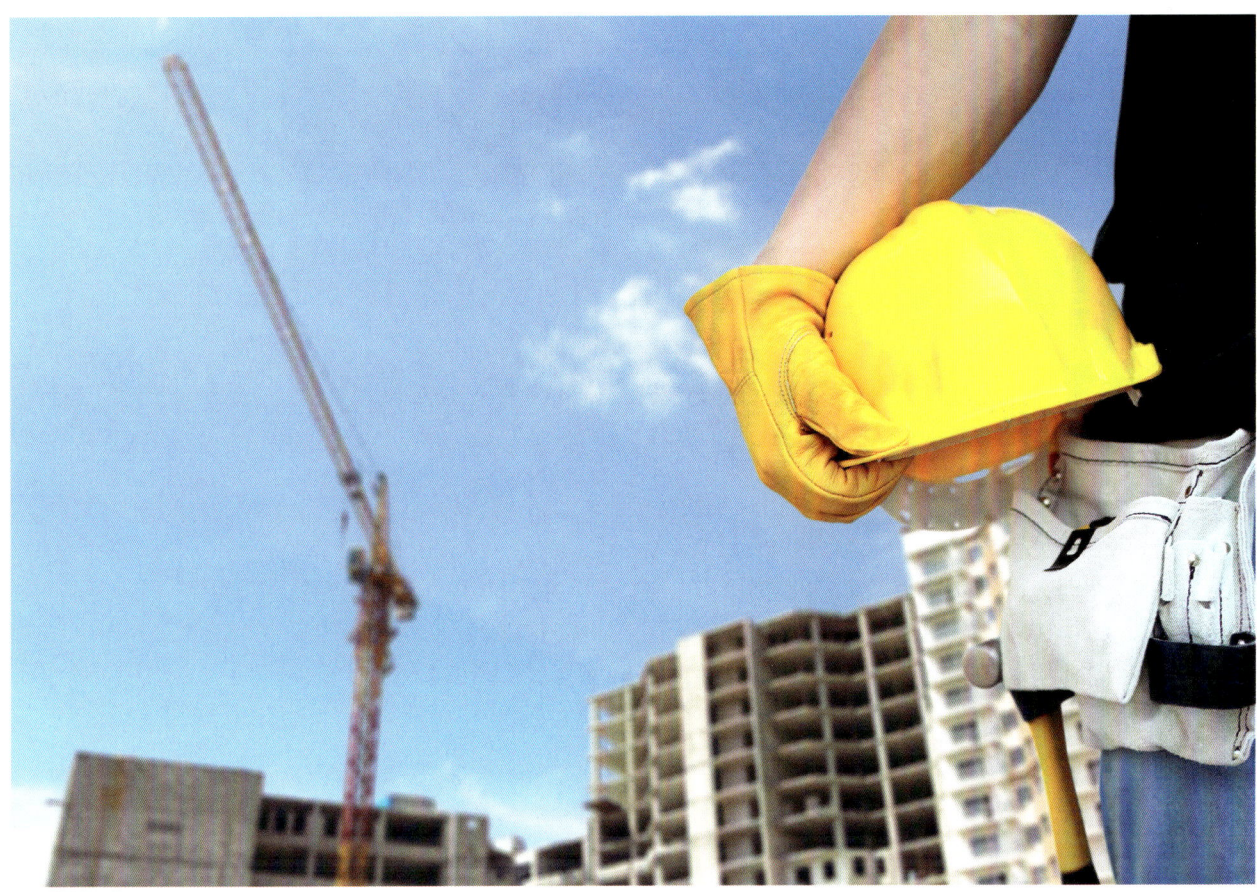

campaigns on alcohol. These efforts should be financed in proportion to their potential impact. The redesigning should be based on needs assessments that are themselves derived from the results of public surveys on alcohol. The redesigned educational programmes should provide information on the risks of alcohol use, the availability and effectiveness of advice and treatment in reducing harmful alcohol use, and the evidence for effective alcohol policies.

Efforts should be made to support and help build the capacity of local communities and municipalities. Increasingly, local communities and municipalities are taking on a wider range of responsibilities to reduce the harmful use of alcohol. This requires increased locally generated training, capacity-building and support of local action groups to ensure that the full range of potential evidence-based policies and actions are put to their full use at the local level.

Community and workplace resources for action on alcohol should be developed. These resources should include documentation of effective alcohol programmes and an analysis of the factors that contribute to success in the community and in the workplace. They should also include assessment tools, so that alcohol programme managers can ensure that these factors are incorporated into the design and implementation of community and workplace programmes.

A mechanism to evaluate and document programmes should be created and financed, in order to strengthen the design and implementation of both new and established programmes, and to achieve the best results in the community and in the workplace.

Relevant national legislation should be revised with a view to its potential amendment, to ensure that it facilitates and supports community and workplace initiatives, rather than hindering them.

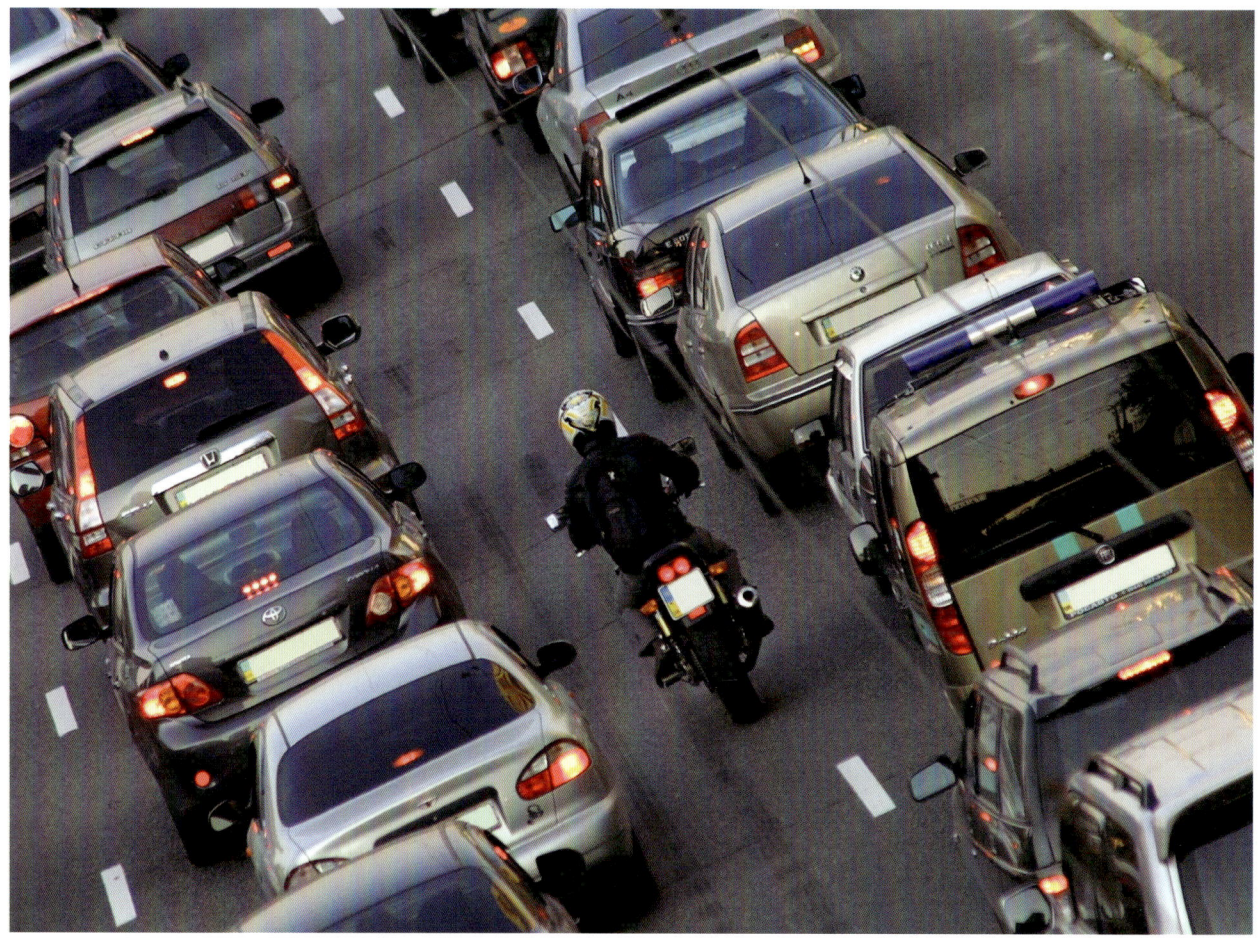

Drink–driving policies and countermeasures

Headline

Even small amounts of alcohol can impair the ability to drive, and action to reduce drinking and driving receives widespread public support, particularly since many of the victims of drink–driving are not the drink–drivers themselves. To be effective in reducing the unnecessary tragedy of drink–driving injuries and fatalities requires sustained joined-up action between government, traffic police, the criminal justice system, safety authorities, the health sector, local communities and other stakeholders.

Outcome

Throughout the duration of this action plan, countries should progressively reduce, and maintain at as low a level as possible, drink–driving fatalities.

Indicator

The indicator for this section would be drink–driving fatalities.

Background

In general, drink–driving fatalities and accidents have been declining in most European countries, although there remains considerable room for improvement. Although young people are at the greatest relative risk of having a drink–driving accident, in absolute terms drink–driving and related accidents and fatalities are more common among the middle-aged. Most Europeans support tougher measures to reduce drink–driving, including greater enforcement by the police. Drink–driving laws, enforcement levels and sanctions might also need to consider the growing number of private and professional drivers who cross borders within the European Region. Repeated offences or very high blood alcohol levels can be an indicator of alcohol use disorders and alcohol dependence, for which treatment should be systematically made available.

Strategies

Action on drinking and driving, and indeed action on the use of other psychoactive substances and driving, reduces the risk of harm not only to the driver but also to passengers, pedestrians and other drivers. One effective intervention is simply to reduce the legal blood alcohol content (BAC) limit for driving, and the effectiveness of this can be heightened if it is part of a combination of other measures. For any country with a BAC limit above 0.5 g/l, it could be beneficial to reduce the level to 0.5 g/l, while countries with a level of 0.5 g/l could benefit from reducing it to 0.2 g/l. However, a lower legal blood alcohol level is only effective if combined with other measures and if it is actually enforced. The best method of enforcement is intelligent random breath-testing that raises the fear of being caught by those who drink and drive rather than in the driving population at large, followed by sobriety checkpoints. Enforcement should be supplemented by public education campaigns to ensure that the public knows the consequences of being apprehended. Enforcement also works best when punishment has severe personal consequences, e.g. on-the-spot fines, driving licence penalty points and, as appropriate, driving licence suspension. It can be further reinforced by court-mandated interventions and the use of alcohol ignition locks for specified periods. Such locks can also be used as a preventive measure, notably for professional drivers.

Options for action

Very few countries would not benefit from lowering their existing BAC limits or improving enforcement. Failure to do so may miss an opportunity to reduce preventable deaths and injuries among drink–drivers and others. There are two particularly important actions that can be taken.

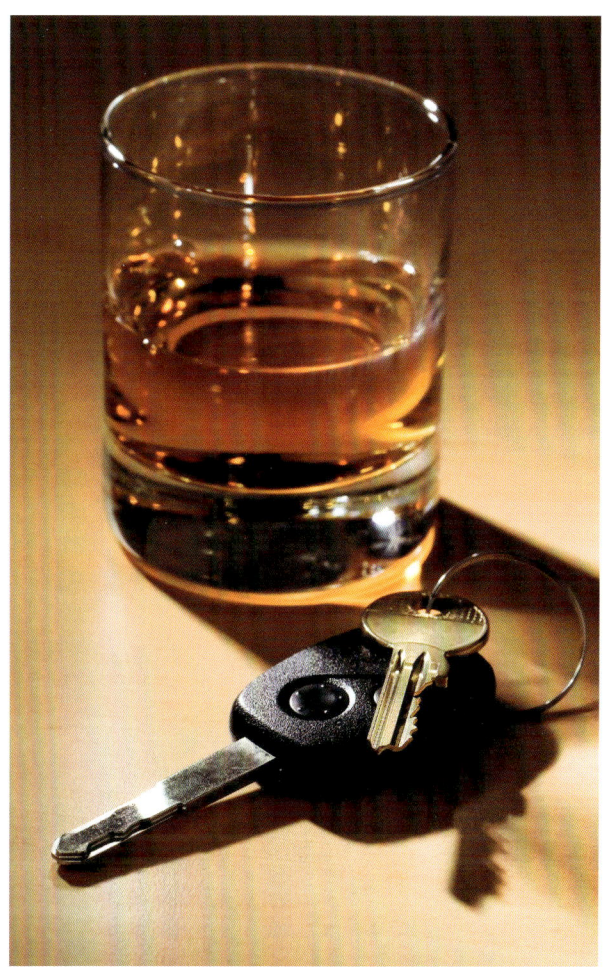

- Reduce the legal BAC level for drinking and driving for all drivers. Whatever the present legal blood alcohol level, evidence suggests that more lives can be saved by reducing it closer to 0.2 g/l. This action sends a basic message and helps to establish "no drinking and driving" as a cultural norm. To be effective, however, a lower BAC limit must be part of a combination of other measures and must be backed up by enforcement.
- Enhance enforcement, either through increased random breath-testing or measures to increase the fear of being caught among those who drink and drive rather than among the driving population at large, or greater use of sobriety checkpoints. In order for BAC limits to be effective, the drink–driver, rather than the driving public, needs to know that there is a real risk of being stopped and breath-tested at any time.

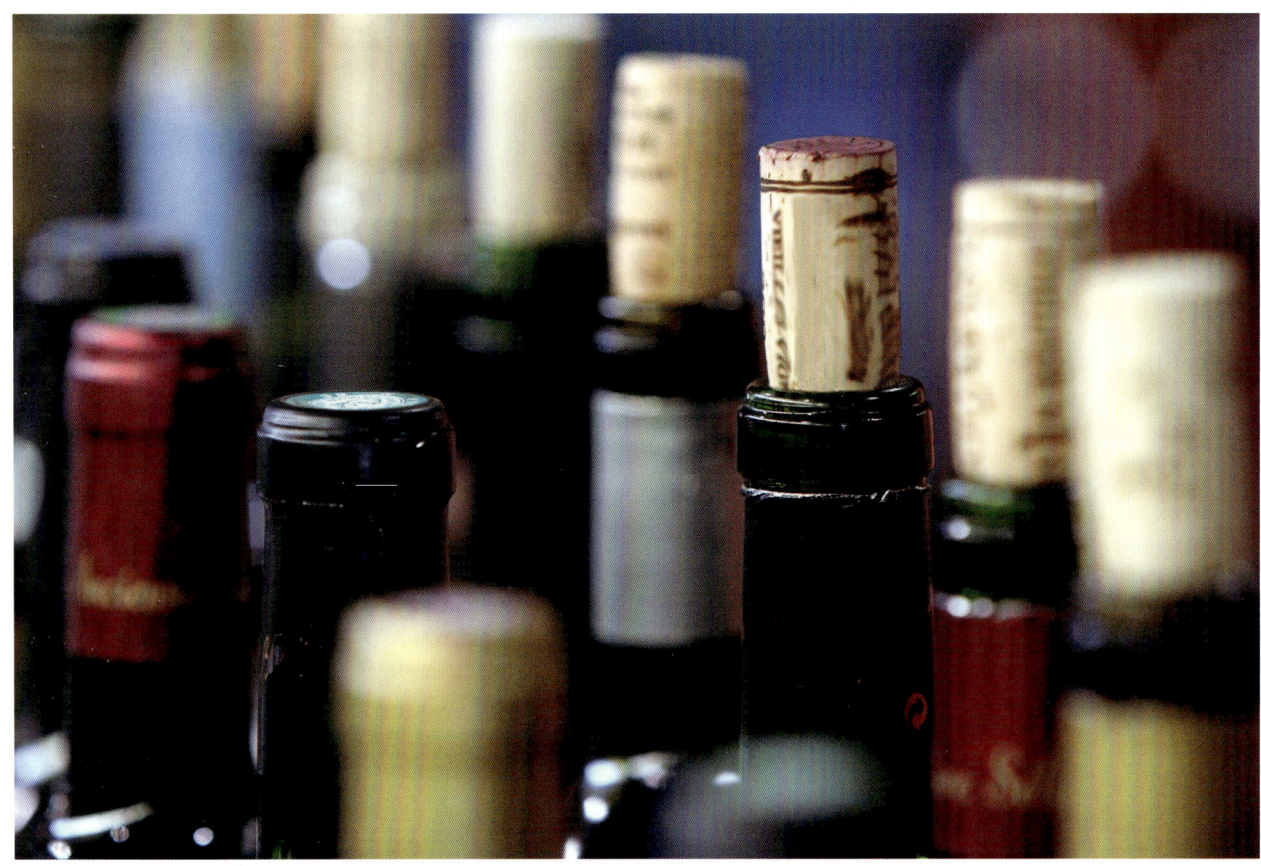

Availability of alcohol

Headline

Studies show that the more available alcohol is, the more it is consumed and the greater the harm that results. The implementation of even small reductions in the availability of alcohol can bring health gain and reduce violence and harm to people other than the drinker. To achieve this requires concerted action between the national authorities, licensing officers, the police, criminal justice systems and the health care sector.

Outcomes

Throughout the duration of this action plan, countries should, where appropriate, limit or reduce the availability of alcohol and ensure that regulations on limiting the sale of alcohol to intoxicated and underage customers are increasingly enforced by all involved parties.

Indicators

Indicators would include a composite measure of alcohol availability, including an assessment of the number of outlets, size and density of outlets, and the days and hours of sale. Underage access to alcohol would also be measured by regular surveys of young people (for example the European School Survey Project on Alcohol and Other Drugs – ESPAD).

Background

A system of licensing for the sale of alcohol enables governments to manage the availability of alcohol, since it allows the government to restrict the number of licences and require licensees to meet certain standards, revoking the licence as a penalty for infringement. While strictly limiting the availability of alcohol may encourage the development of a parallel market in illicit alcohol, it can usually be controlled through enforcement. Another way to reduce harm is to impose situational bans on the use of alcohol in particular locations (such as parks, streets, hospitals and workplaces) and circumstances (such as during football matches). A few countries maintain government monopolies on alcohol sales, which tend to mean fewer stores and shorter opening hours than in countries with private sales.

Strategies

Encouragement should be given in all Member States to introducing or maintaining licensing systems for alcohol sales. Licences may only be renewed for establishments that adhere to laws restricting sales to underage drinkers and intoxicated people, and that discourage patrons from being a public nuisance or engaging in violence. Licensing authorities should be more closely involved in designing, and where appropriate, implementing measures aimed at reducing alcohol-related incidents of violence, crime, public disturbance and harm to health. Those countries with government monopolies for the retail sale of alcohol should consider preserving them.

Governments should take steps to control the availability of alcohol where necessary, such as by regulating the density of alcohol outlets and controlling the sales hours. It is advisable to avoid extending the days and hours of alcohol sales, and to curtail them further when given neighbourhoods or communities experience excessive alcohol-related harm. Minimum purchase ages for alcohol should be enforced. Where they are less than 18 years, it would be advantageous to increase them to 18 for all beverage products in both off-trade and on-trade establishments. Efforts could be envisaged to control implementation, such as using young test buyers to ensure that establishments enforce minimum purchase ages.

Options for action

Most jurisdictions provide opportunities to control the sale of alcohol in ways that can reduce alcohol-related harm, notably through better enforcement. Enforcement appears to be a major deficiency in European alcohol efforts, particularly the enforcement of minimum age laws and laws against selling alcohol to already intoxicated customers. It is also worthwhile to review ways to control the density and sale hours of alcohol outlets by strengthening existing laws and regulations. A wide range of options is available.

- If the minimum purchase age is less than 18 years, consideration should be given raising it to 18 years for all beverage categories, including beer and wine, at all sales outlets, including supermarkets, bars and cafes. Countries with higher age limits than 18 years for buying alcohol products should not lower these.
- Strengthen existing laws and regulations to reduce the density and opening hours of alcohol sales outlets, and, where they exist, maintain a government retail monopoly.
- Mount educational and legislative efforts to increase enforcement of bans on selling alcohol to people under legal age.

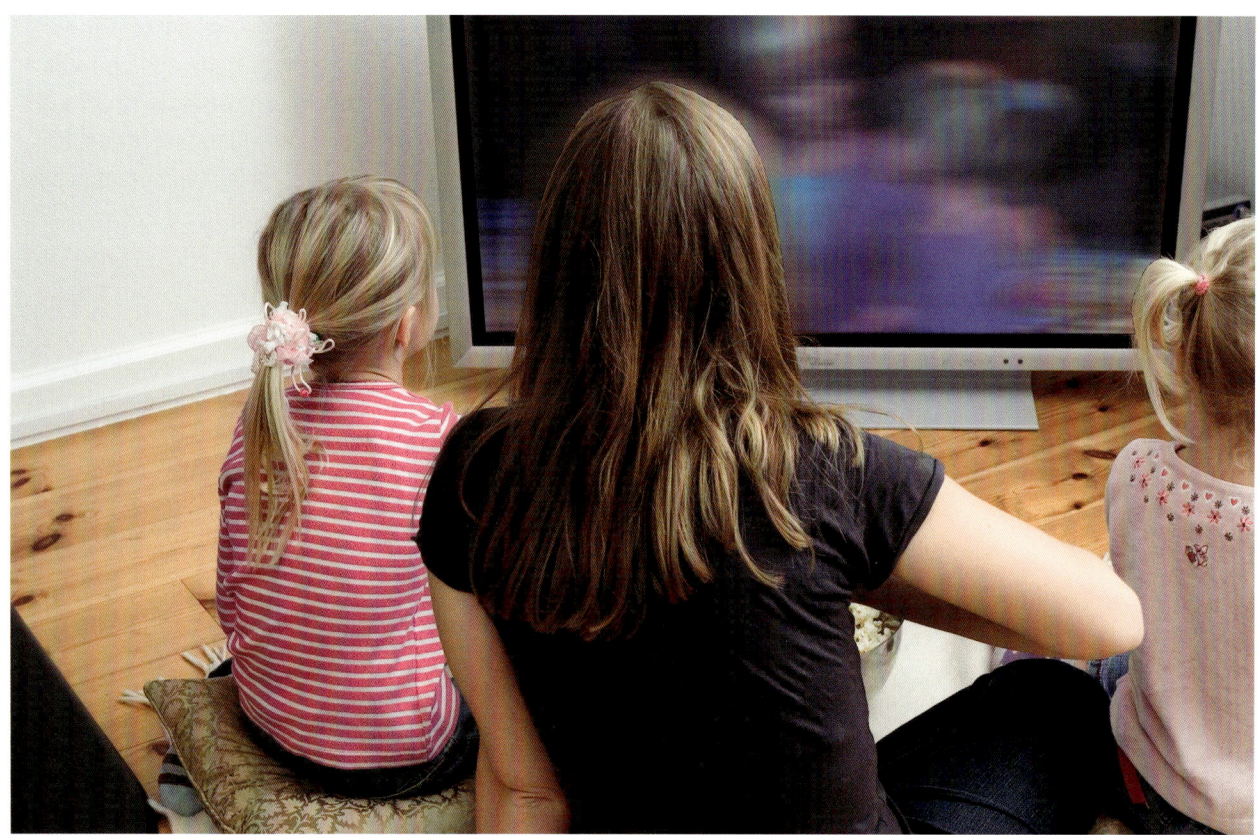

Marketing of alcoholic beverages

Headline

The extent and breadth of commercial communications on alcohol and their impact, particularly on young people's drinking, should not be underestimated. There are many ways to limit exposure to commercial communications, ranging from avoiding the use of humour and glamour and other youth-appealing aspects, to avoiding sponsorship and television and cinema advertising, all the way up to a complete ban. Whatever system is adopted, joint work between government, health systems, the media and all forms of telecommunications is essential. More than this, international coherence is needed, since communications cross borders.

Outcome

Throughout the duration of this action plan, and in particular to protect children and young people, countries should have systems in place to prevent inappropriate and irresponsible alcohol advertising and marketing that targets children and young people.

Indicator

The indicator here would be children's and young people's reported exposure to the full range of alcohol marketing, assessed using surveys conducted every one or two years and also taking into account other drivers of behaviour.

Background

The marketing of alcohol is an enormous activity in itself, and continues to expand through different communication channels. A full marketing strategy includes not only advertising and promotional activities, but also product development, price-setting and targeting different market segments with different products. Moreover, alcohol is no longer marketed only through traditional broadcast media (such as television and radio) and traditional non-broadcast media (such as print media, billboards and branded merchandise). It is also promoted by linking alcohol brands to sports and cultural activities through sponsorship and product placement, and by direct marketing using technologies such as the Internet, podcasts and text messaging. In addition, the entire entertainment sector plays a role in shaping the expectations of young people for the use of alcohol through its portrayal of alcohol in films, television shows, songs and other cultural productions. Accordingly, any effort to regulate irresponsible alcohol marketing should be comprehensive and address all these elements. Finally, given that commercial communications cross borders, international action is needed.

Strategies

Both the content of alcohol marketing and the amount of exposure to it are critical issues for young people, who are particularly susceptible to alcohol's harmful effects. Young people's interest in specific aspects of marketing materials, such as humour, animation and popular music, contributes significantly to the materials' overall effectiveness. Studies show that there is a dose–response relationship between young people's exposure to alcohol marketing and the likelihood that they will start to drink or drink more.[6] Real-time studies have shown that marketing can have an immediate and substantive impact on how much young people drink, and that this impact is even greater on heavier drinkers.

Although many jurisdictions regulate the volume and content of alcohol advertisements, their regulations may not always reflect sufficient knowledge of how young people respond to advertising and the aspects of advertising they are drawn to. Many forms of marketing exposure often remain unregulated, for example the portrayal of alcohol use in films, product placement in films and on television shows, and advertising on the Internet and through mobile communication devices. Some jurisdictions have restricted certain forms of alcohol marketing, such as prohibiting it from television and cinemas or forbidding sports sponsorships.

In some jurisdictions, the content and placement of alcohol marketing is controlled through systems of co-regulation and self-regulation by economic operators, including advertisers, the media and alcohol producers. To be effective, however, such regulation requires a clear framework and sufficient incentives to succeed. Monitoring of alcohol marketing practices is best done when it is the responsibility of an independent body or a government agency, and when it is performed systematically and routinely. Because it can be quite difficult for advertising codes or laws to specify all aspects that should not be permitted in alcohol advertising, some countries (France) have chosen to specify what it can include, since that is much clearer to monitor and enforce.

Options for action

The impact of marketing on the use and heavy use of alcohol should not be underestimated. Systems for managing the marketing of alcohol can be made more efficient, reducing exposure for the benefit of public health. Given the cross-border nature of commercial communications on alcohol, supranational action is also needed. Possible actions are mentioned below:

- setting up regulatory or co-regulatory frameworks, preferably with a legislative basis and supported when appropriate by self-regulatory measures, for alcohol marketing by:
  – regulating the content and volume of marketing;
  – regulating sponsorship activities that promote alcoholic beverages;
  – restricting or banning promotions in connection with activities targeting young people;
  – regulating new forms of alcohol marketing techniques, for instance social media;
- development by public agencies or independent bodies of effective systems of surveillance of marketing of alcohol products;
- setting up effective administrative and deterrence systems for infringements of marketing restrictions;
- regulating direct or indirect marketing in some or all media.

---

[6] Anderson P et al. Impact of alcohol advertising and media exposure on adolescent alcohol use: a systematic review of longitudinal studies. *Alcohol and Alcoholism*, 2009, 44(3):229–243.

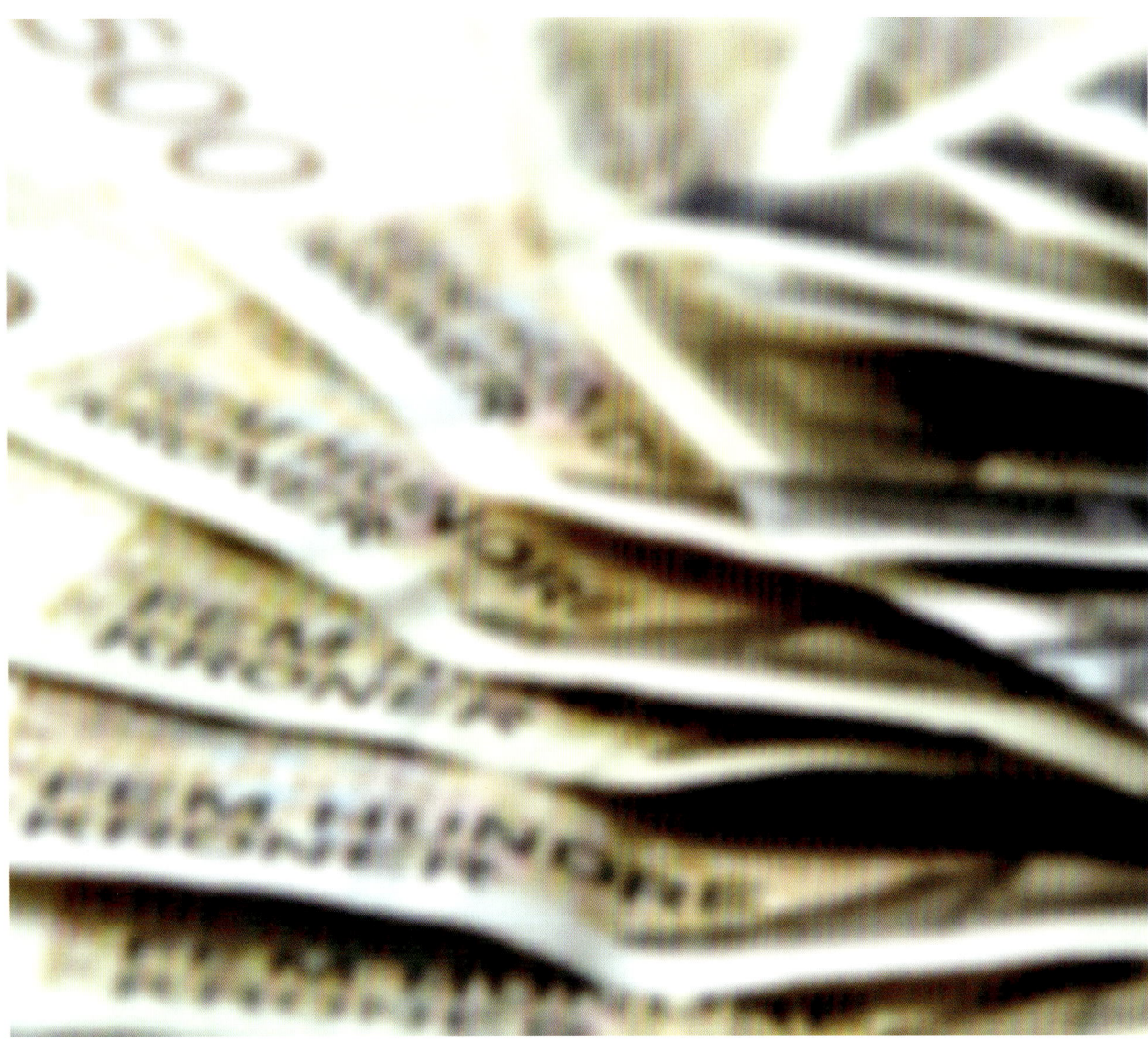

Pricing policies

Headline

When other factors are held constant, such as income and the price of other goods, a rise in alcohol prices leads to reduced alcohol consumption and reduced alcohol-related harm, and vice versa. Price increases correlate with a reduction in the harm caused by alcohol, which also indicates that heavier drinking has been reduced

Taxes are one way to influence the price of alcohol, with immediate and greater impact on heavier drinkers. Strong relationships are needed between health departments (ministries) and tax departments (ministries) to make the continued case that tax may be able to play a role in reducing the harmful use of alcohol.

Outcome

Throughout the duration of this action plan, countries should include pricing policies as part of a comprehensive strategy.

Indicator

The indicator in this case would be the affordability of alcohol (measured by comparing the relative alcohol price index against the real household disposable income index).

Background

Of all alcohol policy measures, the evidence is strongest for the impact of alcohol prices as an incentive to reduce heavy drinking occasions and regular harmful drinking. The gains are greatest for younger and heavier drinkers and for the well-being of people exposed to the heavy drinking of others.

Strategies

Alcohol taxes must address a number of objectives, and reducing the harmful use of alcohol is a factor that countries should consider when setting their tax rates. Increased taxes do not necessarily mean increased prices, since alcohol producers and retailers can offset tax increases by not passing on the tax increase to the consumer. One way to manage this is to introduce a legal minimum price per litre of alcohol. It can be argued that light drinkers are punished by tax increases and that governments will consider the impact on this group seriously. However, it can also be argued that raising taxes or introducing a minimum price hardly affects the alcohol consumption and out-of-pocket expenses of light drinkers. It is also possible to restrict the use of direct and indirect price promotions, discount sales, sales below cost and flat rates for unlimited drinking or other types of volume sales. Reductions in the damage that drinkers inflict on others may also benefit light drinkers. While it has also been argued that tax increases cause job losses, in fact the long-term effects of higher alcohol taxes on employment as a whole are likely to be neutral, with less unemployment if anything, although there may be some short-term adjustments in the hospitality sector. One of the main determinants of alcohol consumption and alcohol-related harm is affordability, a composite measure of the price of alcohol relative to the price of other goods, adjusted for income. In order to protect public health, alcohol taxes may need to be adjusted to ensure that alcohol does not become

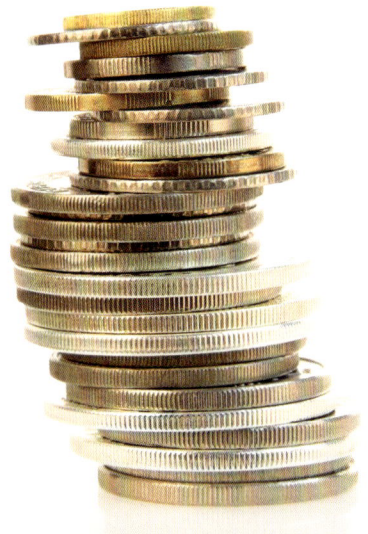

more affordable. The existence of a substantial illicit or informal market for alcohol can complicate the policy considerations for alcohol taxes. In such circumstances, tax increases should be accompanied by government efforts to control these markets. Cross-border trade can also complicate policy considerations for alcohol taxes, although it is important to note that decreasing taxes tends to lead to more alcohol-related harm rather than resolving cross-border issues.

Options for action

In most countries, leaving alcohol taxes unchanged would mean that the relative price of alcohol falls, with a consequent rise in heavy drinking occasions, alcohol-related harm and lower productivity. Taking into account that it is a sovereign right of the Member States to determine and establish their taxation policies, the possible options for actions are:

- to increase alcohol taxes: elasticity and affordability data can inform the extent to which alcohol tax should be increased;
- to institute proportionally higher taxes on products with a higher alcohol concentration or incentives on lower-alcohol versions of products;
- to add special taxes to products that are especially attractive to young consumers; several countries have instituted such taxes for alcopops and related beverages;
- to establish a minimum price per litre of pure alcohol; in countries that choose this option, this measure may be more likely to ensure that price changes result in a desired change in the retail price, which tax increases may circumvent if they are not passed on to the consumer.

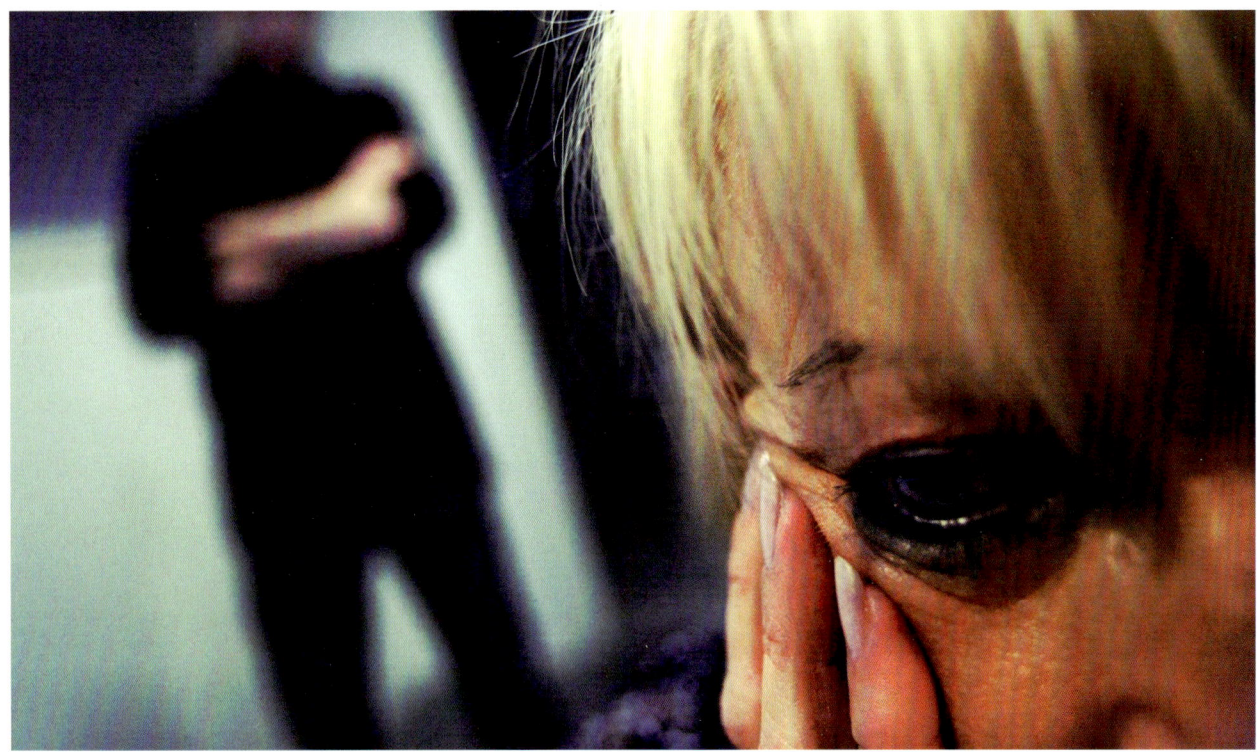

Reducing the negative consequences of drinking and alcohol intoxication

Headline

Most alcohol is consumed in heavy drinking patterns, and this is the most risky form of drinking, which harms people other than the drinker and can cause considerable harm to drinkers themselves, not only through accidents and sudden death but also death from long-term chronic conditions. All policy options proposed in this action plan are likely to reduce the frequency and size of heavy drinking patterns, but action in drinking environments is also fundamentally important. To be effective, this requires a coordinated response between government, health systems, the police, criminal justice systems, licensing authorities, retailers and alcohol outlets, local communities and other stakeholders.

Outcome

Throughout the duration of this action plan, countries should tackle death rates as a consequence of alcohol intoxication, and in particular alcohol-related intentional and unintentional injuries.

Indicator

Death rates from alcohol-related intentional and unintentional injuries will be the indicator for this section.

Background

Heavy drinking occasions and intoxication that can occur in all settings, including the home as well as drinking outlets, are particularly harmful to health and social well-being. While all action areas in this plan can impact on heavy drinking, this action area focuses on the consequences of intoxication that result from drinking environments. The ready availability of cheap alcohol from other retail outlets may result in many customers arriving at drinking environments already intoxicated. Nevertheless, drinking environments can be associated with drunkenness, drink–driving and aggressive and violent behaviour, and some premises are associated with a disproportionate amount of harm. The relationship between drinking and alcohol-related harm can be both affected and mediated by the physical and social context of drinking. Interventions in drinking environments can be important in averting problems that often harm people who are not drinking, notably the problems of drink–driving and violence.

Strategies

Bars are one important part of the drinking environment. Elements of bar environments that increase the likelihood of alcohol-related problems include serving practices that promote intoxication, aggressive enforcement of closing time by bar staff and local police, the inability of bar staff to manage problem behaviour, characteristics such as crowding, and a willingness to serve underage or intoxicated individuals. Adherence to bar policies for preventing intoxication has resulted in only modest reductions in heavy consumption and higher-risk drinking. Impact is greatly enhanced, however, when there is active, continual enforcement of laws prohibiting the sale of alcohol to intoxicated customers. For those countries that do not have one, introducing a licensing system for the sale of alcohol, and regulations for the issuance of licences, can ensure that serving establishments meet certain standards to decrease the likelihood of alcohol-related harm. These regulations can be monitored regularly at the local level and sanctions imposed for violating them, including loss of licence. Server training programmes could be a prerequisite for receiving and maintaining a licence.

Health warning labels should be placed on all alcoholic beverage containers as part of broader communication and point-of-purchase health campaigns to reduce the harmful use of alcohol. Once phased in, alcohol warning or information labels cost very little and, at the very least, remind consumers and society at large that alcohol is no ordinary commodity. In line with the provision of information on ordinary foodstuffs, alcoholic beverage labels should state the alcohol content in an easily understood manner and state the Member State's guidelines for men and women. The ingredients relevant to health, including the calorie content, should be listed and in general labelling should be introduced like that used for other foodstuffs, in order to ensure that consumers have access to complete information on the content and composition of the product for the protection of their health and interests.

Options for action

Since all jurisdictions are likely to have serving establishments with poorly designed premises or that violate laws against serving underage or intoxicated customers, there is always room to step up such efforts at the local level to reduce harm. Important actions can be taken in that regard.

Guidelines and standards could be developed for the design of serving premises, server training and monitoring and enforcing licensing laws. These could be disseminated among licensing authorities and serving establishments. These guidelines and standards could reflect a public health orientation.

Existing licensing regulations should be reviewed and strengthened where appropriate. The regulations should ensure that serving premises meet established standards, that server training is considered for licensing, that the regulations are regularly monitored and enforced at a local level, that there are sufficiently severe sanctions (including licence revocation) for violations by servers or serving establishments, and that there are sufficiently severe sanctions for licensing bodies that fail to regulate drinking environments effectively.

Measures could be taken to introduce a series of warning or information labels on all alcoholic beverage containers and on all commercial communication materials for alcoholic beverages. The content of the messages can usefully be advised by public health bodies. The focus of such messages might be to address issues of immediate concern such as drinking during pregnancy or while driving, or to cover the long-term risks of alcohol use, such as high blood pressure and cancer.

Product labelling similar to that used for foodstuffs, including alcohol and calorie content, additives, allergens etc, can be introduced where possible.

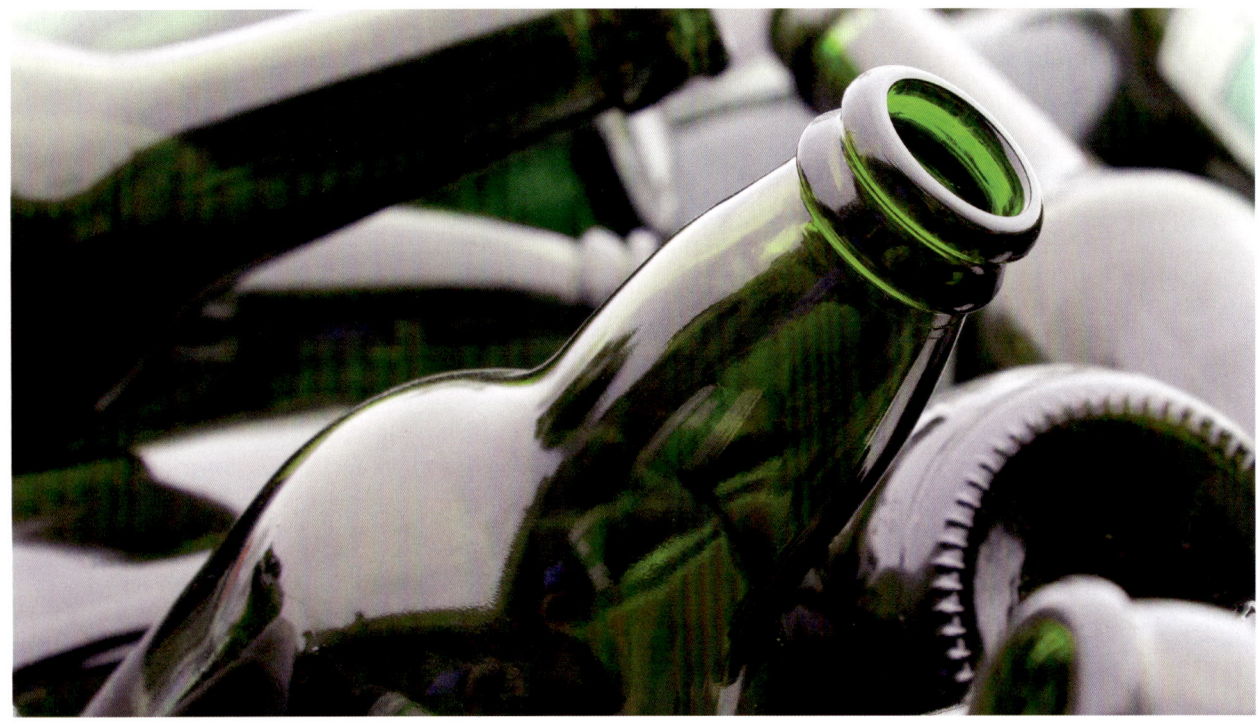

Reducing the public health impact of illicit alcohol and informally produced alcohol

Headline

Throughout Europe, although the exact amount of unrecorded alcohol consumed is not fully known, estimates suggest that overall it could be as high as between one third and two fifths, being much higher in the eastern part of the Region than in the western part. Per unit of alcohol, unrecorded alcohol is considered to have a greater impact on health than recorded alcohol, although the size of this potential problem is not known. The focus of alcohol policy should be to reduce the harm from recorded alcohol and to bring more unrecorded alcohol into the recorded and managed system, while at the same time undertaking a full assessment of the extent of potential harm from all forms of unrecorded alcohol.

Outcome

Throughout the duration of this action plan, countries with an identified problem should reduce the harmful chemical composition of unrecorded alcohols.

Indicator

The acetaldehyde, coumarin, phthalate and ethyl carbamate content of samples of unrecorded alcohols would serve as indicators in this case.

Background

The term "unrecorded alcohol" covers informal and homemade alcohols, illegally-produced or smuggled alcohol products, as well as surrogate alcohol that is not officially intended for human consumption. Illegally- and informally-produced alcohol and surrogate alcohol can have health consequences when consumed owing to their higher ethanol content or contamination, which are toxic to the liver. Illegally traded alcohol can also pose health risks due to its lower cost, which encourages higher consumption, particularly among young and underage people.

Strategies

Despite concerns about potential health harms from the chemical composition of unrecorded alcohol, there are surprisingly few data on the problem in the European Region. A small study of samples collected from 17 European countries found that although samples frequently had higher ethanol concentrations than in recorded spirits, most were generally free of contaminants. The exceptions were fruit spirits, which tended to have high levels of ethyl carbamate. Alcohol policy currently includes no evidence-based concept for managing unrecorded alcohol, with the exception of some successful past policy measures, including the prohibition of methanol to denature alcohol. Additional measures might range from legalizing unrecorded alcohol with subsequent quality control, to instructing the producers of unrecorded alcohol on how to avoid the problems detected.

Although any heavily taxed product will be susceptible to fraudulent activity, that does not mean that reduced, uniform tax rates will reduce the level of alcohol smuggling. Two tools that could help monitor and combat smuggling are the computerization of surveillance data on the movement of excise products, and the issuance of tax stamps to show when and where duty is paid.

Options for action

The main focus of alcohol policy should continue to be on reducing the harm done by recorded alcohol. Nevertheless, there remains a lack of knowledge about the extent of illegal trade and the potential health impact of unrecorded alcohol. Additional health gains can be achieved through a number of actions.

Steps should be taken to make new estimates of the size of the illegal market, and extensive chemical testing of samples of unrecorded alcohol should be conducted to identify the riskiest products and their potential for harm.

Where appropriate, work should be carried out with manufacturers of informal or surrogate products to reduce the risk of harm from manufacturing processes. Computerized tracking should be used to monitor the movement of alcoholic products, and tax stamps should be introduced to facilitate the tracking and identification of illicit products.

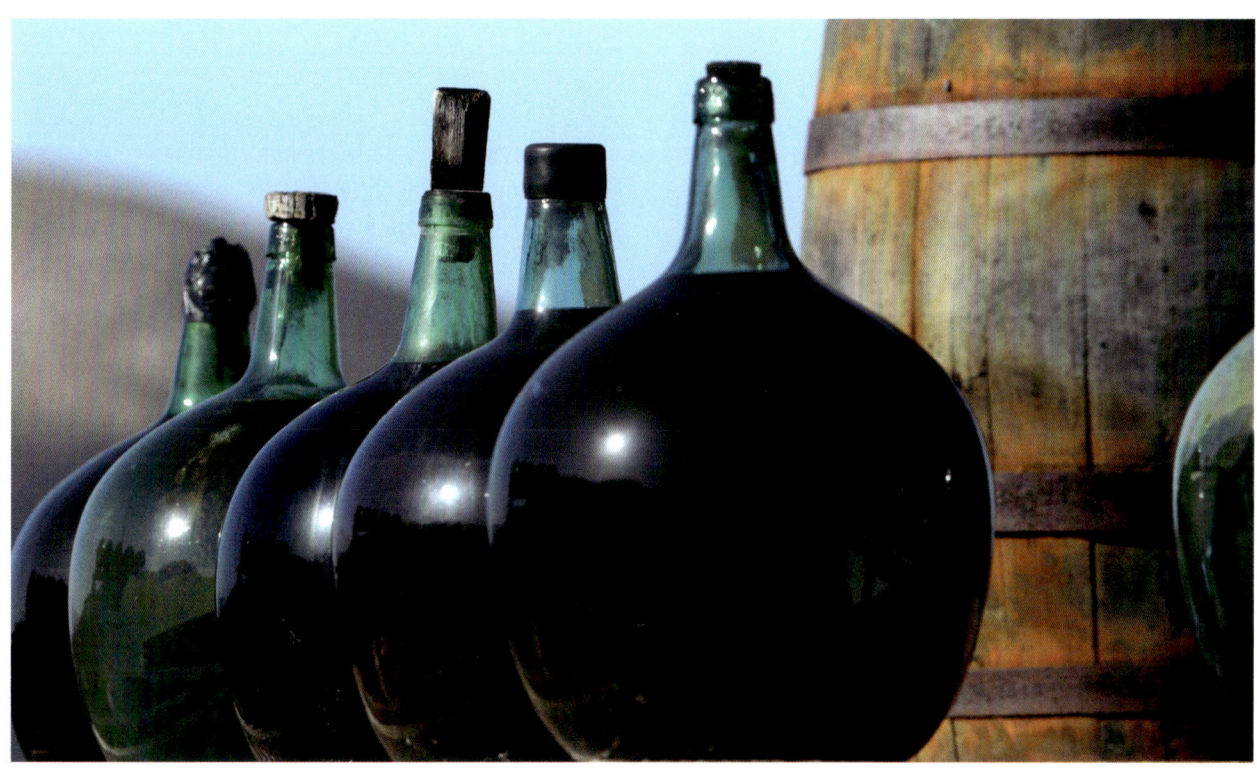

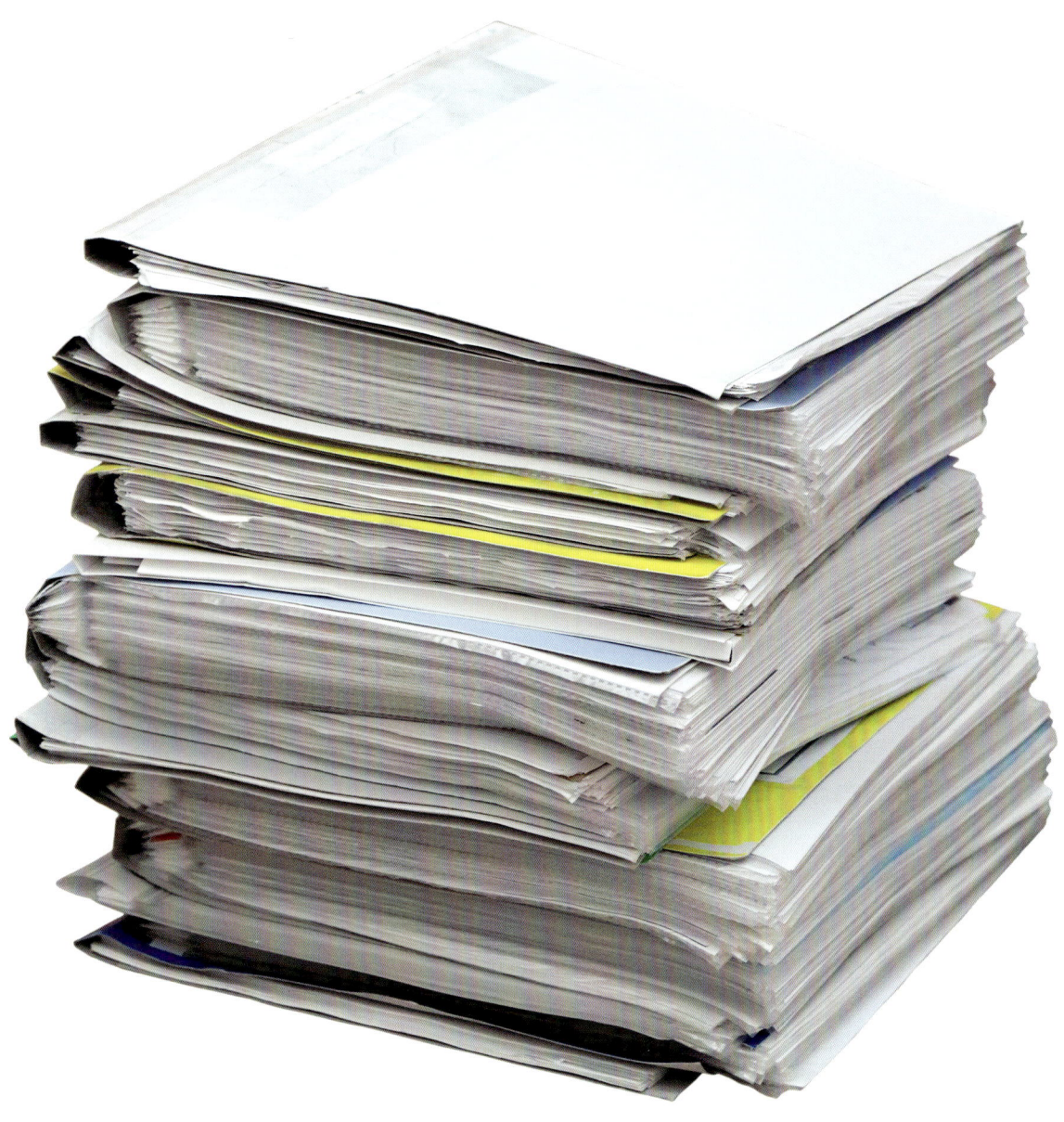

Monitoring and surveillance

Headline

An action plan is more effective if its implementation and impact in reducing alcohol-related harm are monitored and evaluated. This requires transparency and regular public reporting on progress. It also requires considerable leadership and adequate resources to ensure that the necessary data are available, and that many different government departments and sectors work together to produce regular and in-depth monitoring and surveillance reports.

Outcome

Countries should publish regular comprehensive reports on alcohol that include information on drinking among adults, underage drinking, drinking-related ill health and costs to society. Countries should present data for all the indicators of the WHO survey on alcohol and health.

Indicator

Public accessibility of regular comprehensive reports on alcohol would be the indicator in this case.

Background

As emphasized in the section on policy response, in order to be effective, national alcohol action plans and strategies should include objectives and outcomes that are publicized and worked towards. Process and outcome indicators should be developed, used and monitored, with regular reports to keep stakeholders informed. Regular evaluation allows tracking of progress in implementing the national action plan or strategy, helps identify what is working and what is not, and enables regular revision of the plan or strategy. The national instrument and monitoring reports should be made public, and public government sectors, NGOs and other stakeholders should be invited to provide comments and feedback on them at regular intervals.

Strategies

The European Commission's Committee on Alcohol Data Collection, Indicators and Definitions has recommended three key indicators for monitoring changes in alcohol consumption and alcohol-related harm. These indicators measure:

- *volume of consumption* (total recorded and unrecorded per capita consumption of pure alcohol in litres by adults (15 years and older), with sub-indicators for beer, wine and spirits);
- *harmful consumption pattern* (intake of at least 60 g of alcohol on a single occasion at least once per month during the previous 12 months); and
- *health harm* (years of life lost – YLL) attributable to alcohol, with sub-indicators for alcohol-attributable YLL from chronic disease and injury).

Regular reports on alcohol can be prepared and cover the following five topics:

- *drinking among adults*, including trends in alcohol consumption, types of alcohol consumed, socioeconomic variables, demographic characteristics, drinking and pregnancy, adults' drinking behaviour and knowledge of alcohol, and geographical patterns of alcohol consumption;
- *underage drinking*, including trends in alcohol consumption, types of alcohol consumed, socioeconomic variables and drinking among different ethnic groups, associations with other substance use, and drinking behaviour and knowledge of alcohol;
- *drinking-related ill health*, including hazardous, harmful and dependent drinking, consultations about drinking with health professionals, alcohol-related hospital admissions and alcohol-related mortality;
- *availability and affordability of alcohol*;
- *costs to society*, including expenditure on alcohol-related harm, alcohol-related crime and alcohol-related traffic accidents; and
- *policy responses*, including all the policy outcomes of this action plan relevant to a country related to leadership, awareness and commitment, health services' response, community and workplace action, drink–driving, availability, marketing, pricing, reducing intoxication, and reducing the impact of illicit and informally produced alcohol.

Options for action

Although a number of countries produce regular reports on alcohol that include collecting all the relevant data, it is likely that countries can find ways to improve these data and strengthen their analytical and reporting systems. Moreover, it is difficult to improve existing action plans and strategies in the absence of a good system for monitoring and evaluation. In that regard, a number of actions would be necessary.

- Assemble all the available data on alcohol in one report covering consumption, harm, social costs and policy responses, and publicize the report widely. This report could also include on rotating basis more detailed information on a given topic.
- Refine the analytical methods used in generating data on alcohol. Morbidity and mortality data should include the calculation of alcohol-attributable fractions. It is also important to estimate the social costs, particularly the avoidable social costs, which result from implementing specific alcohol policy measures.

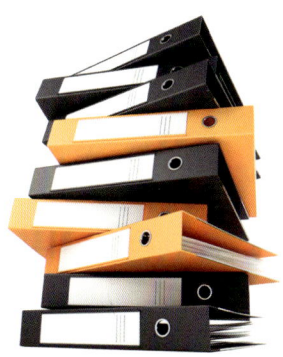

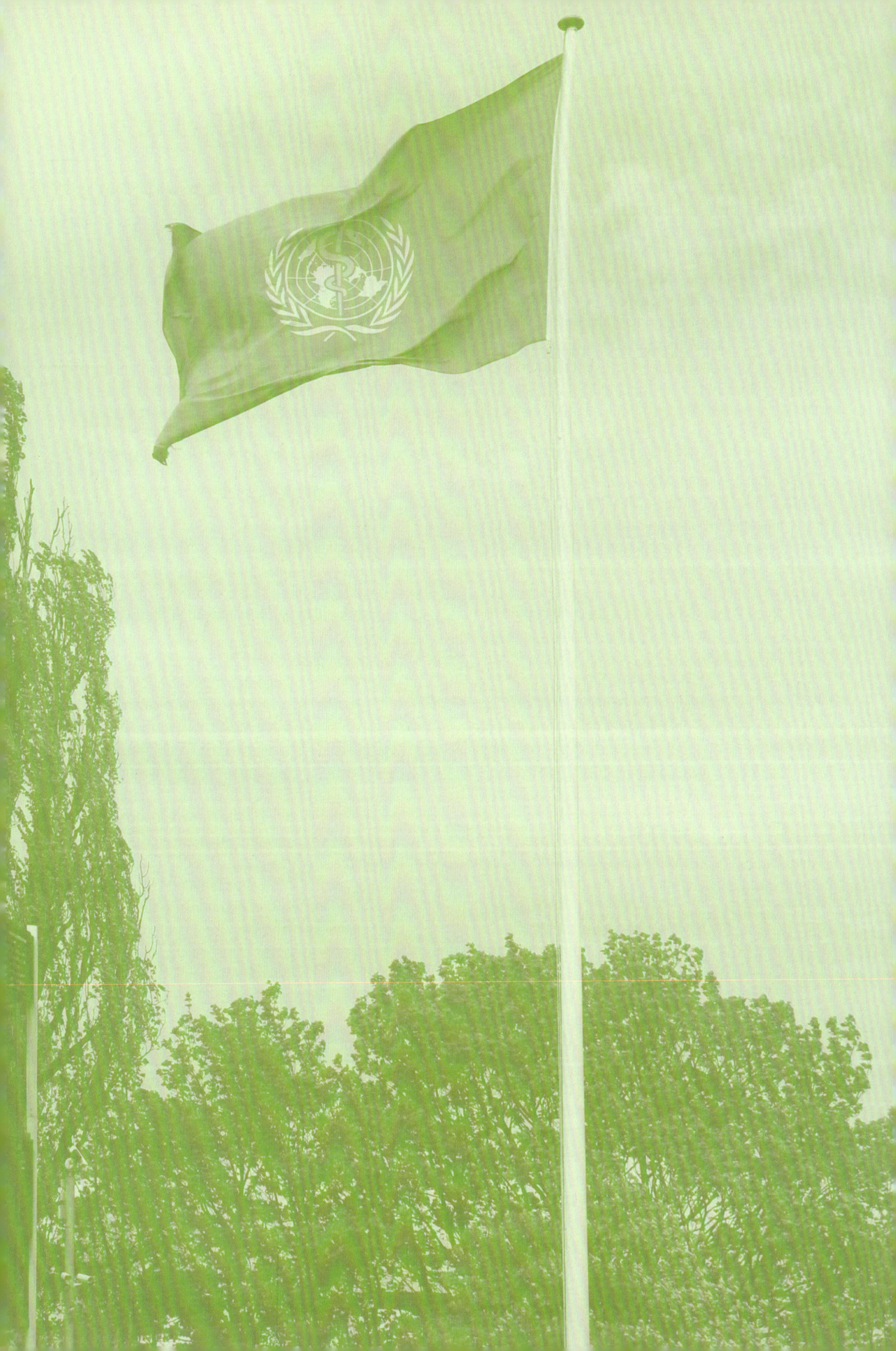

Role of the WHO Regional Office for Europe

Leadership

The WHO Regional Office, together with its collaborating centres, will continue to play a leading role in coordinating a European response to the particular challenges of alcohol-related harm in Europe. The Regional Office will work closely with WHO headquarters to support the European and global implementation of the global strategy to reduce the harmful use of alcohol.

The Regional Office will use the action plan for a publication that will include a checklist or set of questions for Member States and an annex where the proposed indicators are operationalized and linked to the indicators used in the European Information System on Alcohol and Health. The Regional Office will continue its close collaboration with the European Commission implementing common and joint actions. The Regional Office will assist countries in the implementation, evaluation and monitoring of alcohol policies, according to their needs, culture and socioeconomic make-up. It will liaise with appropriate intergovernmental agencies such as the United Nations Development Programme, the World Bank, the International Labour Organization, the World Trade Organization and the Organisation for Economic Co-operation and Development, to seek the inclusion of alcohol policies in relevant social and economic development agendas.

Capacity-building

Within the context of a public health approach to alcohol-related problems, the Regional Office will support government bodies at national and subnational levels, and in particular in those countries with the highest burden of alcohol-related disability and death, to give high priority to preventing the harm done by alcohol, with an increased investment in the implementation of policies known to be effective. The Regional Office will support countries in continuing to review the nature and extent of the problems caused by alcohol in their populations, the resources and infrastructures available for reducing their incidence, prevalence and impact, and the opportunities and possible constraints in establishing new policies and programmes. It will also support countries' efforts to formulate, develop and implement adequately financed action plans on alcohol with clear objectives, strategies and targets, and to establish or reinforce mechanisms and focal points to coordinate the work of public health stakeholders. Furthermore, the Regional Office will assist Member States in implementing and evaluating evidence-based policies and programmes, utilizing existing structures where feasible.

Monitoring and surveillance

In view of the need to provide a sustainable system for monitoring and surveillance of progress in reducing the harmful consequences of alcohol use, the Regional Office will continue, in partnership with the European Commission and WHO headquarters, to maintain and further develop the European Information System on Alcohol and Health, with country-based counterparts, to bring together and analyse alcohol monitoring and surveillance information based on agreed and established comparable data and definitions. The Regional Office will support the integration of relevant data from international agencies such as the European Commission into this system, to allow continuation of current monitoring efforts as well as to provide information for countries that have not yet established an alcohol monitoring and surveillance system. WHO will encourage all stakeholders to provide transparent data and information on issues relating to alcohol.

The Regional Office will continue the function of integrating policies, laws and regulations and data on the effectiveness of policies and programmes into the information system, to help identify best practices and support the Member States in shaping effective programmes.

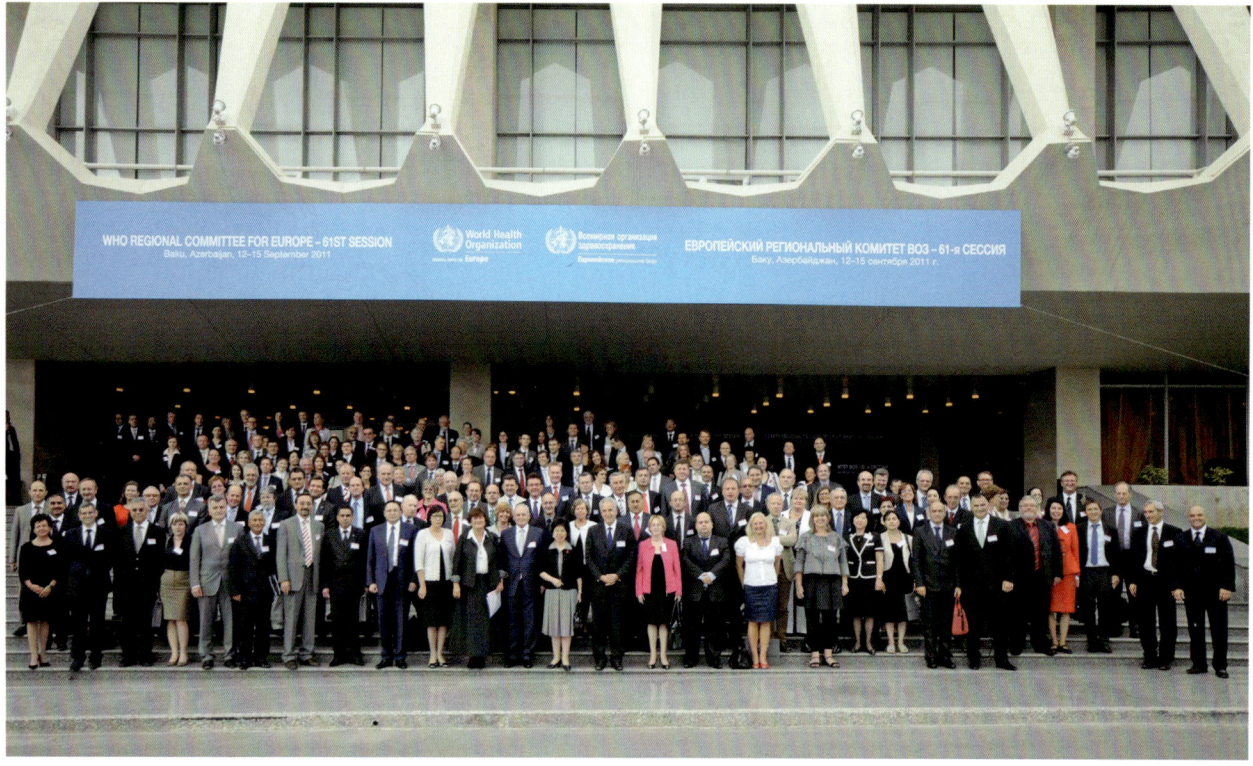

Knowledge dissemination

In order to take advantage of the large and growing body of knowledge, and to sustain and implement evidence-based measures to reduce the harmful use of alcohol, the Regional Office will use its best efforts to communicate with Member States on a regular basis new findings on evidence-based alcohol policy measures and their implementation, and will establish a function to document, collate and disseminate practical experiences with the implementation of evidence-based alcohol policies in different societal circumstances and at different levels of governance.

Working with others

Recognizing the role that NGOs can play in supporting alcohol policy, the Regional Office will strengthen its processes of consultation and collaboration with NGOs and relevant professional bodies that are free of conflicts of interest with the public health interest.

The Regional Office is guided by the principle that public policies and interventions to prevent and reduce alcohol-related harm should be guided and formulated by public health interests and based on clear public health goals and the best available evidence.

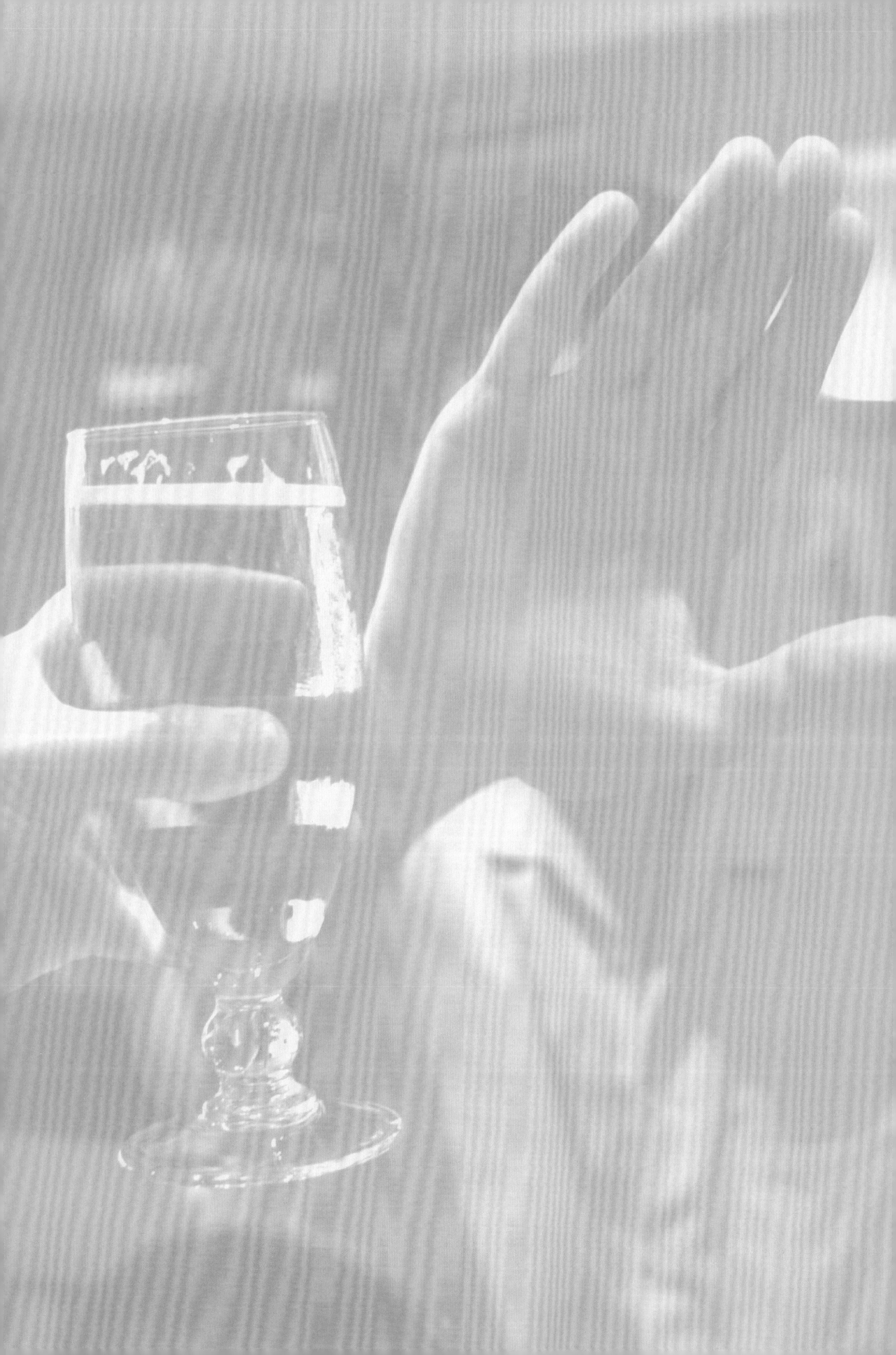

Annexes

The text of WHO Regional Committee for Europe resolution EUR/RC61/R4 on the European action plan to reduce the harmful use of alcohol 2012–2020 is in Annex 1.

With the adoption of the action plan, the Regional Office was requested to produce a publication containing the text of the action plan and the following two new annexes:

- a list of the proposed indicators, with definitions, linked to the indicators used in the European Information System on Alcohol and Health[1] (Annex 2); and
- a checklist or set of questions for Member States (Annex 3).

The Regional Office was also requested to consult Member States when the annexes were prepared and before the document was published. The comments from Member States have been incorporated into the final annexes.

The indicators were drawn from existing sources, including the European Information System on Alcohol and Health[1] and the European Health for All database.[2] Where the European and the global indicators are the same, the definitions developed by WHO headquarters and available in the *Indicator code book*[3] have been used.

The annexes should be viewed as a tool to support Member States in the implementation, evaluation and monitoring of individual national alcohol policies. All indicators are voluntary and not all of them may be relevant for all Member States. Furthermore, the list is not intended to be comprehensive, and Member States may find it appropriate to develop additional indicators according to their needs.

---

[1] European Information System on Alcohol and Health [online database]. Geneva, World Health Organization, 2011 (http://apps.who.int/ghodata/?theme=GISAH&region=euro, accessed 16 October 2012).

[2] European Health for All database (HFA-DB) [online database]. Copenhagen, WHO Regional Office for Europe, 2012 (http://data.euro.who.int/hfadb/, accessed 16 October 2012).

[3] *Indicator code book. Global Information System on Alcohol and Health*. Geneva, World Health Organization, 2012 (http://www.who.int/substance_abuse/activities/gisah_indicatorbook.pdf, accessed 16 October 2012).

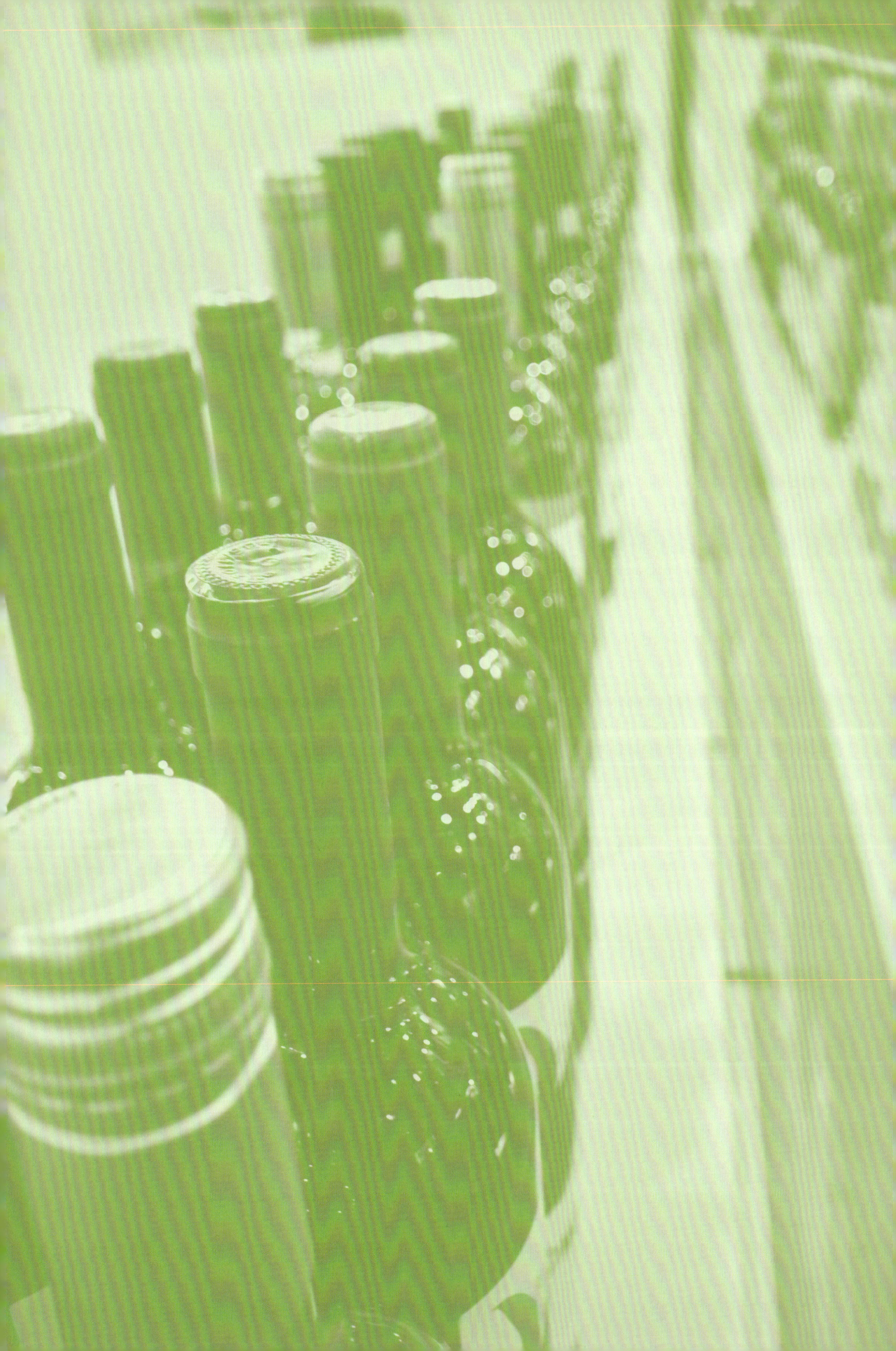

Annex 1
WHO Regional Committee for Europe resolution EUR/RC61/R4

European action plan to reduce the harmful use of alcohol 2012–2020

The Regional Committee,

Reaffirming that the harmful use of alcohol is a major public health concern, with the highest levels of consumption and harm in the WHO European Region;

Recalling its resolution EUR/RC42/R8, by which it approved the first and second phases of the European alcohol action plan, and the European Charter on Alcohol adopted at the European Conference on Health, Society and Alcohol in Paris in December 1995;

Recalling its resolutions EUR/RC49/R8, by which it approved the third phase of the European alcohol action plan, and EUR/RC51/R4 by which it endorsed the Declaration on Young People and Alcohol adopted at the WHO Ministerial Conference on Young People and Alcohol in Stockholm in February 2001;

Recalling World Health Assembly resolution WHA58.26 on public health problems caused by harmful use of alcohol;

Recalling its resolution EUR/RC55/R1, by which it approved the Framework for alcohol policy in the WHO European Region;

Recalling World Health Assembly resolutions WHA61.4 on strategies to reduce the harmful use of alcohol and WHA63.13 on a global strategy to reduce the harmful use of alcohol;

Having considered the European action plan to reduce the harmful use of alcohol 2012–2020;[1]

Affirming that the action plan aims to give guidance about action to fight alcohol-related harm at all levels and to set priority areas for European action, for increased international cooperation and for the participation of all Member States in a cost–effective, appropriate and comprehensive response that takes due account of religious and cultural diversities;

Recognizing that the action plan will be in line and coordinated with the European Action Plan on Noncommunicable Diseases 2012–2016, the Framework for action on public health and Health 2020, the new European policy for health;

Recognizing the threats posed to public health by the harmful use of alcohol and the importance of ensuring that in implementing the action plan, Member States seek the support and engagement of all the sectors involved in a multidisciplinary approach;

Aware that public health concerns regarding the harmful use of alcohol need to be duly considered in the formulation of economic, marketing and trade policy at national and international levels;

Acknowledging the leading role of WHO in promoting international collaboration for the implementation of effective and evidence-based alcohol policies;

1. AGREES that the European action plan to reduce the harmful use of alcohol 2012–2020 offers guidance and policy options for Member States in the WHO European Region, taking into account existing commitments as well as new developments, challenges and opportunities for national and international action;

---

[1] Document EUR/RC61/13.

2. RECOMMENDS Member States:[2]
   (a) to use the action plan to formulate or, if appropriate, reformulate national alcohol policies and national alcohol action plans;
   (b) to strengthen international collaboration in the face of increasing levels of common and transboundary challenges and threats in this area;
   (c) to promote and support policies and interventions to decrease the harmful use of alcohol that preserve and protect public health interests while ensuring that measures to this effect remain proportionate and evidence-based;
   (d) to promote an evidence-based approach that includes all levels of government, as well as all affected sectors and stakeholders involved including communities, civil society and the private sector in the actions needed to prevent or reduce alcohol-related harm;
   (e) to promote alcohol-free policies in an increasing number of settings and circumstances such as the workplace, means of public transport, the environments of children and youth and during pregnancy;
   (f) to reduce exposure to alcohol marketing, and in particular to protect children and youth from alcohol marketing of all kinds;
   (g) to ensure, that in doing so, the measures aiming at reducing the harmful use of alcohol comply with international treaties and agreements;

3. CALLS UPON international, intergovernmental and nongovernmental organizations, as well as self-help organizations, to support the action plan and to work jointly with Member States and with the WHO Regional Office to develop and implement national policies to reduce the negative health and social consequences of the harmful use of alcohol;

4. REQUESTS the Regional Director:
   (a) to exercise leadership in tackling this public health problem and support policy-makers in Europe with formulating national policies and plans as part of their overall response to noncommunicable diseases;
   (b) to monitor the progress, impact and implementation of the action plan, use the information collected to revise and update the European Information System on Alcohol and Health, and use data to compile regular progress reports of alcohol consumption, harm and responses in the Region;
   (c) to mobilize resources in order to ensure adequate health promotion, disease prevention, disease management, research, evaluation and surveillance activities in the Region, in line with the aims of the action plan;
   (d) to cooperate with and assist Member States and organizations in their efforts to develop and implement national policies that prevent or reduce the harm resulting from alcohol consumption and alcohol-related harm in the Region;
   (e) to promote partnerships with governmental and nongovernmental organizations and between Member States, as well as with WHO, other international organizations and regional actors in support of thea ction Plan; and
   (f) to mobilize other international organizations in order to pursue the aims of the action plan.

---

[2] And, where applicable, regional economic integration organizations.

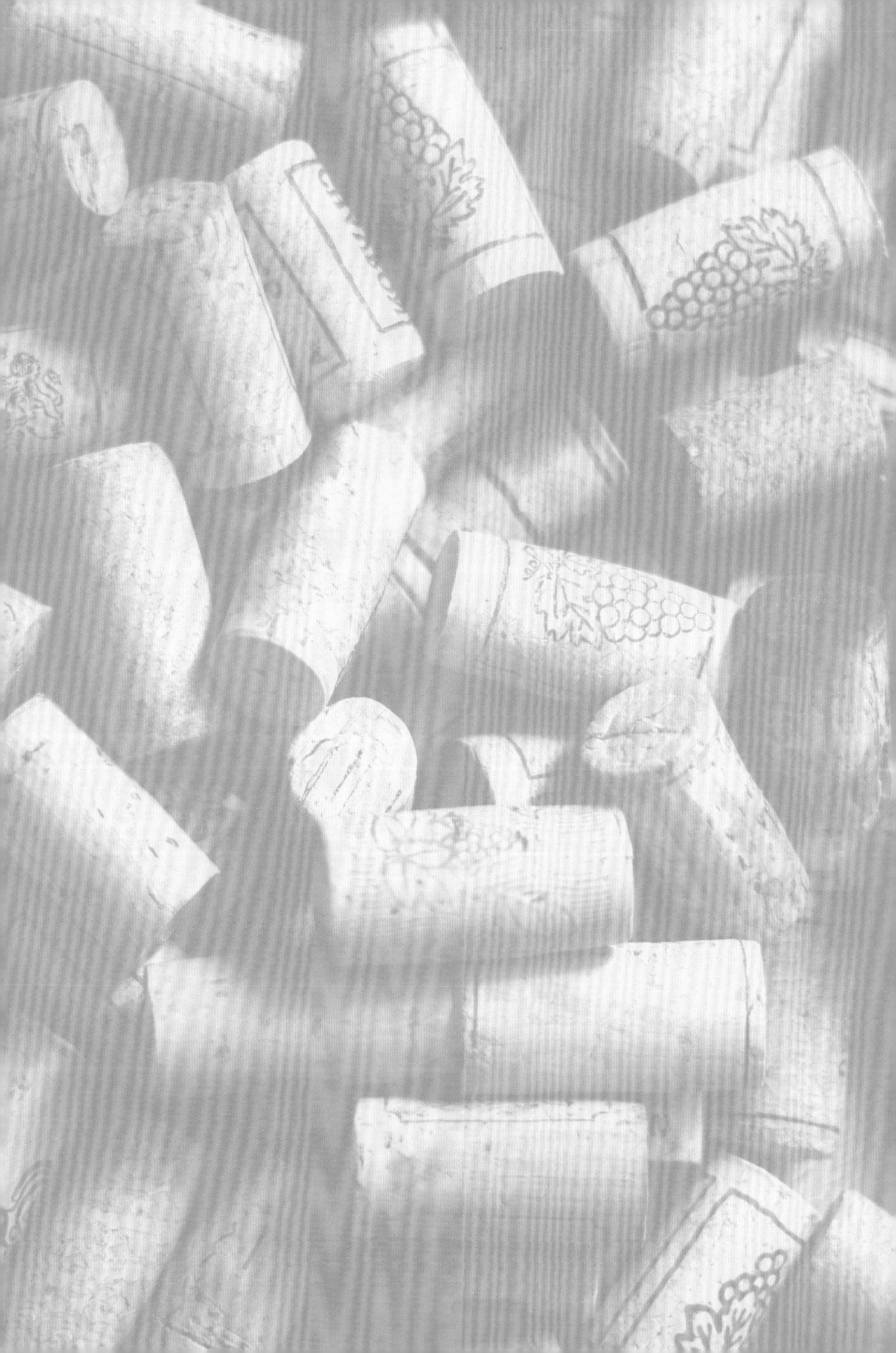

Annex 2
Indicators

Indicators on consumption and harm linked to those in the European Information System on Alcohol and Health

Indicator name	Recorded adult (aged 15+ years) per capita consumption of pure alcohol
Definition	Recorded amount of alcohol consumed per adult (aged 15+ years) over a calendar year in a country, in litres of pure alcohol. The indicator only takes into account the consumption recorded from production, import, export and sales data, often via taxation. Numerator: the amount of recorded alcohol consumed per adult (aged 15+ years) during a calendar year, in litres of pure alcohol. Denominator: midyear resident population (aged 15+ years) for the same calendar year (United Nations World Population Prospects,[1] medium variant). Disaggregated by type of alcoholic beverage.
Data type representation	Rate

Indicator name	Unrecorded adult (aged 15+ years) per capita consumption of pure alcohol
Definition	Unrecorded amount of alcohol consumed per adult (aged 15+ years) in litres of pure alcohol. Unrecorded consumption refers to alcohol which is not taxed and is outside the usual system of governmental control, such as home- or informally-produced alcohol (legal or illegal), smuggled alcohol, surrogate alcohol (not intended for human consumption), or alcohol obtained through cross-border shopping (which is recorded in a different jurisdiction). Numerator: the amount of unrecorded alcohol consumed per adult (aged 15+ years) during a calendar year, in litres of pure alcohol. Denominator: midyear resident population (aged 15+ years) for the same calendar year (United Nations World Population Prospects, medium variant).
Data type representation	Rate

---

[1] World Population Prospects, the 2010 revision [online database]. New York, United Nations, Department of Economic and Social Affairs, Population Division, Population Estimates and Projections Section, 2011 (http://esa.un.org/unpd/wpp/index.htm, accessed 16 October 2012).

Indicator name	Total adult (aged 15+ years) per capita consumption of pure alcohol
Definition	Total (sum of recorded and unrecorded) amount of alcohol consumed per adult (aged 15+ years) over a calendar year, in litres of pure alcohol. Recorded alcohol consumption refers to official statistics (production, import, export, and sales or taxation data), while the unrecorded alcohol consumption refers to alcohol which is not taxed and is outside the usual system of governmental control. In circumstances in which the number of tourists per year is at least the number of inhabitants, the tourist consumption is also taken into account and is deducted from the country's recorded adult per capita consumption.
Data type representation	Rate

Indicator name	Total adult (aged 15+ years) per capita consumption of pure alcohol among drinkers
Definition	Total (recorded and unrecorded) amount of alcohol consumed per adult drinker (aged 15+ years) over a calendar year, in litres of pure alcohol. Numerator: total adult per capita consumption. Denominator: one minus total rate of abstainers.
Data type representation	Rate

Indicator name	Abstainers (aged 15+ years), lifetime
Definition	Proportion of adults (aged 15+ years) in a given population who have not consumed any alcohol during their lifetime, assessed at a given point in time. Numerator: number of lifetime abstainers (aged 15+ years). Denominator: total number of participants (aged 15+ years) responding to the corresponding question in a given survey. Weighted by survey design.
Data type representation	Percentage

Indicator name	Abstainers (aged 15+ years), past 12 months
Definition	Proportion of adults (aged 15+ years) in a given population who have not consumed any alcohol during the past 12 months, assessed at a given point in time. Numerator: number of abstainers (aged 15+ years) in the past 12 months. Denominator: total number of participants (aged 15+ years) responding to the corresponding question in a given survey. Weighted by survey design.
Data type representation	Percentage

Indicator name	Abstainers (aged 18–24 years), lifetime
Definition	Proportion of persons aged 18–24 years in a given population who have not consumed any alcohol during their lifetime, assessed at a given point in time.
Data type representation	Percentage

Indicator name	Abstainers (aged 18–24 years), past 12 months
Definition	Proportion of persons aged 18–24 years in a given population who have not consumed any alcohol during the past 12 months, assessed at a given point in time.
Data type representation	Percentage

Indicator name	Heavy episodic drinkers (binge drinking)
Definition	Proportion of adults (aged 15+ years) who have consumed at least 60 g or more of pure alcohol on at least one occasion weekly. A consumption of 60 g of pure alcohol corresponds to approximately 6 standard alcoholic drinks. Numerator: the (appropriately weighted) number of respondents (aged 15+ years) who reported drinking 60 g or more of pure alcohol on at least one occasion weekly. Denominator: total number of participants (aged 15+ years) responding to the corresponding question(s) in the survey, plus abstainers. Disaggregated by sex.
Data type representation	Percentage

Indicator name	Heavy episodic drinkers among drinkers
Definition	Proportion of adult drinkers (aged 15+ years) who have consumed at least 60 g or more of pure alcohol on at least one occasion weekly over the past year. A consumption of 60 g of pure alcohol corresponds to approximately 6 standard alcoholic drinks. Numerator: the appropriately weighted number of drinkers (aged 15+ years) who reported drinking at least 60 g or more of pure alcohol on at least one occasion weekly. Denominator: total number of respondents (aged 15+ years, appropriately weighted) to the corresponding survey question(s) who reported having consumed an alcoholic standard drink (10 g) within the past 12 months in the same survey.
Data type representation	Percentage

Indicator name	Age-standardized death rates (aged 15+ years) of alcohol-related conditions
Definition	Number of individuals in a given population who died from alcoholic liver disease (ICD-10[2] code K70), liver cirrhosis (codes K70, K74), road traffic accidents (codes V01–V04, V06, V09–V80, V87, V89 and V99), poisoning (codes X40–X49), acts of physical violence (codes X85–Y09, Y871), respectively, during a calendar year. Death rates are age-standardized by the WHO standard population. Numerator: total number of deaths from the respective condition as mentioned above during a calendar year among the country's population. Denominator: whenever available, population data as provided by the countries. In the absence of reported population data, the estimated population data prepared by the United Nations Population Division are used. Deaths are per 100 000 population. Disaggregated by sex.
Data type representation	Rate

Indicator name	Hospital discharges, alcohol-related injuries and poisoning
Definition	Number of persons diagnosed with alcohol-related injuries and poisoning who were treated in hospital and discharged within a calendar year, divided by the total population. Rate per 100 000 population.
Data type representation	Rate

Indicator name	Hospital discharges, alcoholic liver disease
Definition	The number of persons diagnosed with alcoholic liver disease who were treated in hospital and released per calendar year, divided by the total population. Rate per 100 000 population.
Data type representation	Rate

Indicator name	Alcoholic psychosis
Definition	Number of new cases of alcoholic psychosis identified in a defined period, divided by the total population. Rate per 100 000 population.
Data type representation	Rate

---

[2] International Classification of Diseases [web site]. Geneva, World Health Organization, 2012 (http://www.who.int/classifications/icd/en, accessed 19 October 2012).

Indicator name	Alcoholic use disorders (point prevalence)
Definition	Adults (aged 15+ years) who suffer from disorders attributable to the consumption of alcohol (ICD-10 codes: F10.1 Harmful use of alcohol; F10.2 Alcohol dependence) during a given calendar year. Numerator: number of adults (aged 15+ years) with a diagnosis of F10.1, F10.2 during a calendar year. Denominator: midyear resident population (aged 15+ years) over the same calendar year (United Nations World Population Prospects, medium variant). Disaggregated by sex.
Data type representation	Percentage

Indicator name	Road traffic accidents involving alcohol
Definition	Road traffic accidents involving one or more persons under the influence of alcohol. Accidents involving personal injury are included. Accidents with only material damage are not included. Definition of road traffic accident according to the Inland Transport Committee of the United Nations Economic Commission for Europe (ECE). From 2002, the data source is the ECE, Statistics of Road Traffic Accidents in Europe. Rate per 100 000 population.
Data type representation	Rate

Indicator name	Road traffic accidents involving alcohol (drink–driving)
Definition	Number of road traffic accidents in a country in a given year where the driver of at least one car involved has exceeded the legal blood alcohol content (BAC) limit in that country, divided by the total population. Rate per 100 000 population.
Data type representation	Rate

Indicator name	Road traffic accidents involving alcohol, percentage of all traffic crashes
Definition	Number of road traffic accidents in a country in a given year where the driver of at least one car involved has exceeded the legal BAC limit in that country, divided by the number of all traffic crashes.
Data type representation	Percentage

Indicators on leadership, awareness and commitment

Indicator name	Data on alcohol disseminated in national annual report
Definition	Dissemination of data on alcohol in a national annual report. A national annual report refers to a written report issued on a yearly basis by the government including information and data on alcohol consumption, health or social services utilization, availability of resources for alcohol use disorders, economic aspects or any other important information related to alcohol use.
Data type representation	Categorical

Indicator name	Importance of role played by stakeholders
Definition	Level of importance of the role played by stakeholders (nongovernmental organizations, health professionals/health services, academic and research organizations, employer and employee organizations, insurance companies, media organizations, alcohol retailers and HORECA (hotel/restaurant/café) businesses, and alcohol manufacturers) in the areas of: • prevention of underage drinking; • targeted support (information, tools, counselling) for harmful and hazardous drinkers; • prevention of drink–driving; • public policy development to reduce alcohol-related harm. The level of importance is measured by the national authorities of a country as part of the WHO European Survey on Alcohol and Health using the categories "high", "medium", "low" or "no involvement".
Data type representation	Categorical

Indicator name	Budget line for alcohol use disorder treatment
Definition	Availability of a regular source of funds in the annual budget of the government which is allocated for action directed towards treatment and treatment services for alcohol use disorders.
Data type representation	Categorical

Indicator name	Budget line for prevention of alcohol use disorders
Definition	Availability of a regular source of funds in the annual budget of the government which is allocated for action directed towards the prevention of alcohol use disorders and prevention services.
Data type representation	Categorical

Indicator name	Designation of alcohol tax revenues to health services
Definition	Designation of alcohol tax revenues to health services.
Data type representation	Categorical

Indicator name	Publicly-funded alcohol research/monitoring
Definition	Provision of publicly-funded alcohol research/monitoring programmes.
Data type representation	Categorical

Indicator name	Public funds designated for alcohol research/monitoring programmes
Definition	Amount of public funds designated for alcohol research/monitoring programmes (in €).
Data type representation	Count

Indicator name	Adopted written national policy on alcohol
Definition	Adoption of a written national policy on alcohol. An adopted written national policy on alcohol is defined as a written organized set of values, principles and objectives for reducing the burden attributable to alcohol in a population.
Data type representation	Categorical

Indicator name	Existence of operational policy/strategy/action plan/special legislation for alcohol
Definition	Indication as to whether a country has an operational policy, strategy, action plan or special legislation for alcohol.
Data type representation	Categorical

Indicator name	Indicators used to measure achievement of policy goals
Definition	Indicators used to measure the achievement of the goal(s) of the national policy on alcohol.
Data type representation	Categorical

Indicator name	Central coordinating entity for alcohol policy development and monitoring
Definition	Indication as to which sector of the government has the overall coordinating responsibility for the development and monitoring of the national policy on alcohol.
Data type representation	Categorical

Indicator name	Central coordinating entity for alcohol policy implementation
Definition	Whether a country has a central coordinating entity for the implementation of the national policy on alcohol. A central coordinating entity oversees the implementation of each specific area covered by the national alcohol policy.
Data type representation	Categorical

Indicator name	Framework of national alcohol policy
Definition	Framework for presentation of the national policy. The national policy can be a specific alcohol policy or it can be integrated into a substance abuse policy, mental health policy, noncommunicable diseases policy, general public health policy or other policy.
Data type representation	Categorical

Indicator name	Multisectoral alcohol policy
Definition	Presence of a national multisectoral policy on alcohol. The national policy on alcohol is multisectoral if different sectors (such as health, social policy, justice, road safety, education, employment, law enforcement or finance/taxation) are represented in the policy.
Data type representation	Categorical

Indicator name	Sectors represented in national alcohol policy
Definition	The different sectors represented in the national policy on alcohol, which can include health, social policy, justice, road safety, education, employment, law enforcement, finance/taxation or others.
Data type representation	Categorical

Indicator name	Community-based interventions/projects involving stakeholders
Definition	Provision of community-based interventions/projects involving stakeholders.
Data type representation	Categorical

Indicator name	Interventions/projects actively involving young people and civil society
Definition	Provision of interventions/projects actively involving young people and civil society.
Data type representation	Categorical

Indicator name	Steps in the alcohol policy/action plan to involve young people in activities to reduce/prevent alcohol-related harm
Definition	Inclusion in the national alcohol policy (or action plan) of steps to specifically involve young people in activities to reduce or prevent alcohol-related harm.
Data type representation	Categorical

Indicator name	Awareness activities
Definition	Provision of awareness activities pertaining to: harm from alcohol, alcohol and health, alcohol at work, drink–driving, illegal/surrogate alcohol, indigenous peoples, pregnancy and alcohol, social harms, young people's drinking.
Data type representation	Categorical

Indicator name	Consumer information on alcohol and health at points of sale
Definition	Provision of pamphlets and other information pertaining to the harms associated with the use of alcohol.
Data type representation	Categorical

Indicators on health services' response

Indicator name	Brief interventions for health promotion/disease prevention
Definition	Provision of short-term interventions in the form of health promotion or disease prevention activities.
Data type representation	Categorical

Indicator name	Training in screening and brief interventions for alcohol problems
Definition	Provision of training in screening and brief interventions for alcohol problems.
Data type representation	Categorical

Indicator name	Clinical guidelines for brief interventions
Definition	Existence of clinical guidelines for brief interventions which have been approved or endorsed by at least one health care professional body.
Data type representation	Categorical

Indicator name	Heavy episodic drinkers (binge drinking)
Definition	Proportion of adults (aged 15+ years) who have consumed at least 60 g or more of pure alcohol on at least one occasion weekly. A consumption of 60 g of pure alcohol corresponds to approximately 6 standard alcoholic drinks. Numerator: the (appropriately weighted) number of respondents (aged 15+ years) who reported drinking 60 g or more of pure alcohol on at least one occasion weekly. Denominator: the total number of participants (aged 15+ years) responding to the corresponding question(s) in the survey, plus abstainers. Disaggregated by sex.
Data type representation	Percentage

Indicator name	Heavy episodic drinkers among drinkers
Definition	Proportion of adult drinkers (aged 15+ years) who have consumed at least 60 g or more of pure alcohol on at least one occasion weekly over the past year. A consumption of 60 g of pure alcohol corresponds to approximately 6 standard alcoholic drinks. Numerator: the appropriately weighted number of drinkers (aged 15+ years) who reported drinking at least 60 g or more of pure alcohol on at least one occasion weekly. Denominator: the total number of respondents (aged 15+ years, appropriately weighted) to the corresponding survey question(s) who reported having consumed an alcoholic standard drink (10 g) within the past 12 months in the same survey.
Data type representation	Percentage

Indicator name	Persons with alcohol use disorders receiving treatment
Definition	Percentage of persons with alcohol use disorders receiving treatment.
Data type representation	Percentage

Indicator name	Counselling for pregnant women with alcohol problems
Definition	Provision of counselling to pregnant women with alcohol problems.
Data type representation	Categorical

Indicator name	Prenatal care for pregnant women with alcohol or drug problems
Definition	Provision of prenatal care services specifically for pregnant women with alcohol or drug problems.
Data type representation	Categorical

Indicator name	Incidence of fetal alcohol syndrome
Definition	Number of newborns diagnosed with fetal alcohol syndrome (ICD-10 code Q86.0) in a calendar year per 100 000 births.
Data type representation	Rate

Indicator name	Counselling for children in families with alcohol problems
Definition	Provision of counselling to children in families with alcohol problems.
Data type representation	Categorical

Indicators on community and workplace action

Indicator name	Educational programmes involving target groups in the school curriculum
Definition	Provision of programmes targeting children and young people below the legal drinking age to make them aware of the harms associated with the use of alcohol.
Data type representation	Categorical

Indicator name	Legal obligation to include alcohol prevention in the school curriculum/health policies
Definition	A legal obligation for schools to carry out alcohol (or broader alcohol and other substance use) prevention as part of the curriculum or as part of school health policies.
Data type representation	Categorical

Indicator name	Guidelines for prevention/reduction of alcohol-related harm in schools
Definition	Existence of national guidelines for the prevention and reduction of alcohol-related harm in school settings.
Data type representation	Categorical

Indicator name	Prevention/counselling at workplaces for persons with alcohol problems
Definition	Provision of prevention/counselling at workplaces for persons with alcohol problems.
Data type representation	Categorical

Indicator name	Workplace accidents involving alcohol
Definition	Number of workplace accidents in a calendar year where alcohol was involved.
Data type representation	Count

Indicator name	Involvement of social partners in prevention of alcohol-related harm at workplaces
Definition	Involvement of social partners representing employers and employees at national level in action to prevent and address alcohol-related harm at workplaces.
Data type representation	Categorical

Indicator name	Community-based interventions/projects involving stakeholders
Definition	Provision of community-based interventions/projects involving stakeholders.
Data type representation	Categorical

Indicator name	National guidelines for community-based interventions to reduce alcohol-related harm
Definition	Existence of national guidelines for implementing effective community-based interventions to reduce alcohol-related harm.
Data type representation	Categorical

Indicator name	National guidelines for alcohol prevention/counselling at workplaces
Definition	Existence of national guidelines for alcohol problem prevention and counselling at workplaces.
Data type representation	Categorical

Indicator name	Legislation on alcohol testing at workplaces
Definition	Existence of legislation on alcohol testing at workplaces.
Data type representation	Categorical

Indicator name	Strength of action in the policy area of alcohol issues at workplaces
Definition	Strength of action over the past five years in the area of action to address alcohol issues at workplaces rated by the national authorities of a country as part of the WHO European Survey on Alcohol and Health using a seven-point scale ranging from +3 (stronger) to -3 (weaker).
Data type representation	Categorical

Indicator name	Strength of action in the policy area of community action to reduce alcohol-related harm
Definition	Strength of action over the past five years in the area of broad-based community action to reduce alcohol-related harm as rated by the national authorities of a country as part of the WHO European Survey on Alcohol and Health using a seven-point scale ranging from +3 (stronger) to -3 (weaker).
Data type representation	Categorical

Indicators on drink–driving policies and countermeasures

Indicator name	BAC limit when driving a vehicle
Definition	Legal maximum BAC (measured as mass per volume) allowed while driving a vehicle in a country. The BAC limits for the general population, young/novice drivers and professional/commercial drivers, respectively, are indicated.
Data type representation	Count

Indicator name	Road traffic accidents involving alcohol
Definition	Road traffic accidents involving one or more persons under the influence of alcohol. Accidents involving personal injury are included. Accidents with only material damage are not included. Definition of road traffic accident according to the Inland Transport Committee of the United Nations ECE. From 2002, the data source is the ECE, Statistics of Road Traffic Accidents in Europe. Rate per 100 000 population.
Data type representation	Rate

Indicator name	Road traffic accidents involving alcohol (drink–driving)
Definition	Number of road traffic accidents in a country in a given year where the driver of at least one car involved has exceeded the legal BAC limit in that country, divided by the total population. Rate per 100 000 population.
Data type representation	Rate

Indicator name	Road traffic accidents involving alcohol, percentage of all traffic crashes
Definition	Number of road traffic accidents in a country in a given year where the driver of at least one car involved has exceeded the legal BAC limit in that country, divided by the number of all traffic crashes.
Data type representation	Percentage

Indicator name	Death rate for alcohol-related road traffic accidents
Definition	Number of alcohol-related road traffic deaths (where the driver of at least one car involved has exceeded the legal BAC limit) among the total population during a calendar year, divided by the total population. Rate per 100 000 population. Disaggregated by sex.
Data type representation	Rate

Indicator name	Enforcement of drink–driving law by random breath-testing or police checkpoints
Definition	Use of random breath-testing or police checkpoints for enforcement of alcohol laws.
Data type representation	Categorical

Indicator name	Level of enforcement of maximum legal BAC for driving
Definition	Level of enforcement at the national level of the maximum legal BAC for driving scored by the national authorities of a country as part of the WHO European Survey on Alcohol and Health using an 11-point scale ranging from 0 (not enforced) to 10 (fully enforced).
Data type representation	Categorical

Indicator name	Vehicles stopped for roadside stationary random breath-testing, as a percentage of all vehicles
Definition	Number of motorized vehicles (cars, motorcycles, lorries, buses, etc.) stopped each year for roadside stationary random breath-testing at police checkpoints, divided by the number of all motorized vehicles.
Data type representation	Percentage

Indicator name	Awareness activities, drink–driving
Definition	Provision of awareness activities relating to drink–driving.
Data type representation	Categorical

Indicator name	Penalties for drink–driving
Definition	On-the-spot fines, driving licence penalty points and/or licence suspension imposed on drivers for disregarding drink–driving laws.
Data type representation	Categorical

Indicator name	Mandatory driver education for habitual offenders
Definition	Mandatory attendance at driver education classes by habitual offenders against drink–driving laws for a designated period of time.
Data type representation	Categorical

Indicator name	Use of alcolocks for drink–driving offenders
Definition	Use of alcolocks in combination with rehabilitation as an alternative to punishment for drink–driving.
Data type representation	Categorical

Indicator name	Use of alcolocks by transport companies
Definition	Voluntary or obligatory use of alcolocks by public or commercial transport companies.
Data type representation	Categorical

Indicators on availability of alcohol

Indicator name	Age limit for on-premise alcohol service
Definition	Age at which a person can be served alcoholic beverages on premises in a country (that is, alcoholic beverages cannot be served to a person under this age). Disaggregated by type of alcoholic beverage.
Data type representation	Count

Indicator name	Age limit for off-premise alcohol sales
Definition	Age at which a person can be sold alcoholic beverages off premises in a country (that is, alcoholic beverages cannot be sold to a person under this age). Disaggregated by type of alcoholic beverage.
Data type representation	Count

Indicator name	National survey on underage drinkers of alcoholic beverages
Definition	The regular conduct of surveys to collect information on alcohol consumption among underage drinkers of alcoholic beverages (children below the legal age for drinking or being sold or served an alcoholic drink) at the national level. This includes school-based and youth health surveys which include, but are not limited to, the collection of data on alcohol consumption.
Data type representation	Categorical

Indicator name	Underage alcohol users
Definition	Number of underage individuals who have consumed alcohol in their lifetime, divided by all individuals in the age group. Total and disaggregated by sex.
Data type representation	Percentage

Indicator name	Licensing for production and sale of alcoholic beverages
Definition	Partial government control of production and sale of alcoholic beverages. Disaggregated by type of alcoholic beverage.
Data type representation	Categorical

Indicator name	Monopoly of the production and sale of alcoholic beverages
Definition	Government monopoly (full control) of production and sale of alcoholic beverages.
Data type representation	Categorical

Indicator name	Restrictions on times of on- and off-premise sales of alcoholic beverages
Definition	Regulated limitations on the time (hours and days) of sales of alcoholic beverages, both on- and off-premises, in a country. Disaggregated by type of alcoholic beverage.
Data type representation	Categorical

Indicator name	Restrictions on locations of on- and off-premise sales of alcoholic beverages
Definition	Regulated limitations on the locations (places and density) of sales of alcoholic beverages, both on- and off-premises, in a country. Disaggregated by type of alcoholic beverage.
Data type representation	Categorical

Indicator name	Restrictions on on- and off-premise sales of alcoholic beverages during specific events
Definition	Regulated limits on sales of alcoholic beverages, both on- and off-premises, during specific events in a country. Disaggregated by type of alcoholic beverage.
Data type representation	Categorical

Indicator name	Restrictions on off-premise sales of alcoholic beverages at petrol stations
Definition	Regulated limits on off-premise sales of alcoholic beverages at petrol stations in a country. Disaggregated by type of alcoholic beverage.
Data type representation	Categorical

Indicator name	Level of enforcement of on-premise sales restrictions
Definition	Level of enforcement of existing on-premise sales restrictions at national level scored by the national authorities of a country as part of the WHO Global Survey on Alcohol and Health using an 11-point scale ranging from 0 (not enforced) to 10 (fully enforced). Judgement may be based on (statistical) information, expert opinion or other factors.
Data type representation	Categorical

Indicator name	Level of enforcement of off-premise sales restrictions
Definition	Level of enforcement of existing off-premise sales restrictions at national level scored by the national authorities of a country as part of the WHO Global Survey on Alcohol and Health using an 11-point scale ranging from 0 (not enforced) to 10 (fully enforced). Judgement may be based on (statistical) information, expert opinion or other factors.
Data type representation	Categorical

Indicator name	Measures to enhance compliance with age limits
Definition	Level of importance of the following measures for enhancing compliance with age limits: • server training as a requirement of licensing • enforcement by the police or other authorities • monitoring through test purchasing • awareness campaigns directed at servers/sellers • awareness campaigns directed at young people, as rated by the national authorities of a country as part of the WHO European Survey on Alcohol and Health using the categories of "high", "medium", "low" or "not used at all". Judgement is based on expert opinion on the current situation in the country.
Data type representation	Categorical

Indicators on marketing of alcoholic beverages

Indicator name	Restrictions on alcohol advertising
Definition	Legally enforced restrictions on alcohol advertising in a country (the promotion of alcoholic beverages by the alcohol industry through a variety of media): national television, cable television, national radio, local radio, print media, cinemas, billboards, point-of-sale, internet. Disaggregated by type of alcoholic beverage.
Data type representation	Categorical

Indicator name	Restrictions on alcohol product placement
Definition	Legally enforced restrictions on alcohol product placement in a country. Product placement refers to the sponsorship of, for example, TV productions by economic operators if their alcoholic beverage is shown in these productions. Disaggregated by type of alcoholic beverage.
Data type representation	Categorical

Indicator name	Restrictions on sponsorship by the alcohol industry
Definition	Legally enforced restrictions on sponsorship by the alcohol industry of sporting events or events for young people in a country. Sponsorship refers to the support of an event financially or through the provision of products or services as part of brand identification and marketing. Disaggregated by type of alcoholic beverage.
Data type representation	Categorical

Indicator name	Restrictions on the promotion of alcohol sales
Definition	Legally enforced restrictions on the promotion of alcohol sales in a country by, for example, producers (parties and events), retailers (including supermarkets) in the form of sales below cost (for example, two for the price of one, happy hours), or owners of pubs and bars (serving alcohol free). Sales promotion refers to marketing practices designed to facilitate the purchase of a product.
Data type representation	Categorical

Indicator name	Level of restriction on alcohol industry sponsorship and alcohol sales promotion
Definition	Total ban, partial statutory restriction, voluntary agreement/self-regulation or no restriction on sponsorship of sporting and youth events by the alcohol industry and sales promotions by producers. Disaggregated by type of alcoholic beverage. "Partial statutory restriction" means that the restriction applies during a certain time of day or to some events, programmes, magazines, films, etc. "Voluntary agreement/self-regulation" means that the alcoholic beverage industry follows its internal voluntary rules.
Data type representation	Categorical

Indicator name	Level of enforcement of advertising restrictions
Definition	Level of enforcement of existing advertising restrictions at national level scored by the national authorities of a country as part of the WHO Global Survey on Alcohol and Health using an 11-point scale ranging from 0 (not enforced) to 10 (fully enforced). Judgement may be based on (statistical) information, expert opinion or other factors.
Data type representation	Categorical

Indicator name	Level of enforcement of alcoholic beverage industry sponsorship restrictions
Definition	Level of enforcement of existing restrictions on alcoholic beverage industry sponsorship at national level as scored by the national authorities of a country as part of the WHO Global Survey on Alcohol and Health using an 11-point scale ranging from 0 (not enforced) to 10 (fully enforced). Judgement may be based on (statistical) information, expert opinion or other factors.
Data type representation	Categorical

Indicator name	Level of enforcement of restrictions on alcoholic beverage sales promotion
Definition	Level of enforcement of existing restrictions on alcoholic beverage sales promotion by producers, retailers and owners of pubs and bars at national level scored by the national authorities of a country as part of the WHO Global Survey on Alcohol and Health using an 11-point scale ranging from 0 (not enforced) to 10 (fully enforced). Judgement may be based on (statistical) information, expert opinion or other factors.
Data type representation	Categorical

Indicator name	Penalties for violations of advertising/product placement legislation
Definition	Provision of penalties for violations of advertising/product placement legislation.
Data type representation	Categorical

Indicator name	Penalties for violations of sponsorship and sales promotion legislation
Definition	Provision of penalties for violations of sponsorship/sales promotion legislation.
Data type representation	Categorical

Indicator name	Level of restriction on alcohol advertising/product placement
Definition	Existence of a total ban, partial statutory restriction, voluntary agreement/self-regulation or no restriction on: • public service/national TV advertising • commercial/private TV advertising • national radio advertising • local radio advertising • printed newspaper/magazine advertising • billboard advertising • point of sale advertising • cinema advertising • internet advertising • public service/national TV product placement • commercial/private TV product placement. Disaggregated by type of alcoholic beverage. "Partial statutory restriction" means that the restriction applies during a certain time of day or to some events, programmes, magazines, films, etc. "Voluntary agreement/self-regulation" means that the alcoholic beverage industry follows its internal voluntary rules
Data type representation	Categorical

Indicators on pricing policies

Indicator name	Adjustment of excise duty tax for alcoholic beverages
Definition	Adjustment of excise duty tax for alcoholic beverages for inflation.
Data type representation	Categorical

Indicator name	Excise duty per hectolitre
Definition	Average alcohol excise duty tax per hectolitre of beer, wine and spirits (in (in €).).
Data type representation	Count

Indicator name	Non-alcoholic beverages at lower prices
Definition	Requirement to offer non-alcoholic beverages at lower prices.
Data type representation	Categorical

Indicator name	Calculation of excise duty tax by volume/weight
Definition	Use of alcohol volume/weight to calculate excise duty tax.
Data type representation	Categorical

Indicator name	Additional levy on specific products
Definition	Additional levy on specific products that are especially attractive to young consumers (such as alcopops).
Data type representation	Categorical

Indicator name	Minimum pricing
Definition	Existence of a minimum price per litre of pure alcohol.
Data type representation	Categorical

Indicator name	Bans on below-cost selling and/or volume discounts
Definition	Bans on sales below cost and/or on volume sales.
Data type representation	Categorical

Indicator name	Level of restriction on sales promotion
Definition	Existence of a total ban, partial statutory restriction, voluntary agreement/self-regulation or no restriction on: • sales promotion by retailers in the form of sales below cost; • sales promotion by owners of pubs and bars in the form of serving alcohol for free. Disaggregated by type of alcoholic beverage. "Partial statutory restriction" means that the restriction applies during a certain time of day or to some events, programmes, magazines, films, etc. "Voluntary agreement/self-regulation" means that the alcoholic beverage industry follows its internal voluntary rules.
Data type representation	Categorical

Indicators on reducing the negative consequences of drinking and alcohol intoxication

Indicator name	Server training
Definition	Server training provided on a regular basis to bar staff and staff at special events that gives them skills and knowledge about alcohol harm and safe-serving practices.
Data type representation	Categorical

Indicator name	Server training required by national licensing system
Definition	Nationwide server training courses organized on a regular basis as required by the national licensing system.
Data type representation	Categorical

Indicator name	Road traffic accidents involving alcohol
Definition	Road traffic accidents involving one or more persons under the influence of alcohol. Accidents involving personal injury are included. Accidents with only material damage are not included. Definition of road traffic accident according to the Inland Transport Committee of the United Nations ECE. From 2002, the data source is the ECE, Statistics of Road Traffic Accidents in Europe, ECE, Geneva. Rate per 100 000 population.
Data type representation	Rate

Indicator name	Road traffic accidents involving alcohol (drink–driving)
Definition	Number of road traffic accidents in a country in a given year where the driver of at least one car involved has exceeded the legal BAC limit in that country, divided by the total population. Rate per 100 000 population.
Data type representation	Rate

Indicator name	Road traffic accidents involving alcohol, percentage of all traffic crashes
Definition	Number of road traffic accidents in a country in a given year where the driver of at least one car involved has exceeded the legal BAC limit in that country, divided by the number of all traffic crashes.
Data type representation	Percentage

Indicator name	Death rate for alcohol-related road traffic accidents
Definition	Number of alcohol-related road traffic deaths (where the driver of at least one car involved has exceeded the legal BAC limit) among the total population during a calendar year, divided by the total population. Rate per 100 000 population. Disaggregated by sex.
Data type representation	Rate

Indicator name	Death rate for all violence
Definition	Number of deaths from physical violence among the total population during a calendar year (ICD-10 codes X85–Y09, Y871), divided by the midyear resident population for the same calendar year (United Nations World Population Prospects, medium variant). Rate per 100 000 population. Disaggregated by sex.
Data type representation	Rate

Indicator name	Hospital discharges, alcohol-related injuries and poisoning
Definition	Number of persons diagnosed with alcohol-related injuries and poisoning treated in hospital and discharged within a calendar year, divided by the total population. Rate per 100 000 population.
Data type representation	Rate

Indicator name	Health warning labels on alcohol advertising
Definition	Presence of health warning labels with information of the dangers associated with the use of the product.
Data type representation	Categorical

Indicator name	Health warning labels on alcohol containers
Definition	Presence of health warning labels providing information to the buyer of the dangers associated with the use of the product.
Data type representation	Categorical

Indicator name	Product labelling on alcohol products
Definition	Provision of legally required product labels on alcohol products (alcohol and calorie content, additives, allergens, etc.).
Data type representation	Categorical

Indicators on reducing the public health impact of illicit alcohol and informally produced alcohol

Indicator name	Estimates of unrecorded alcohol consumption
Definition	Availability of estimates on unrecorded consumption of alcoholic beverages at the national level.
Data type representation	Categorical

Indicator name	Duty paid or excise stamp on alcohol container
Definition	Use of excise stamps on alcohol containers by national customs to signify that the excise tax has been paid.
Data type representation	Categorical

Indicators on monitoring and surveillance

Indicator name	System for monitoring alcohol-related harm
Definition	Presence of a system for monitoring alcohol-related harm (alcohol-related mortality, alcohol-related morbidity and alcohol-related social consequences).
Data type representation	Categorical

Indicator name	Data collection on alcohol-related health indicators
Definition	Collection of data on alcohol-related health indicators (indicators for those disorders directly or indirectly associated with the use of alcohol).
Data type representation	Categorical

Indicator name	Data collection on recorded adult per capita alcohol consumption
Definition	Collection of data on recorded adult per capita alcohol consumption every year.
Data type representation	Categorical

Indicator name	Estimates of unrecorded alcohol consumption
Definition	Availability of estimates of unrecorded consumption of alcoholic beverages at the national level.
Data type representation	Categorical

Indicator name	National survey of alcohol consumers in the general population
Definition	National surveys of alcohol consumption in the general population.
Data type representation	Categorical

Indicator name	National survey of abstainers
Definition	National surveys of rates of abstainers (for example, lifetime, past year) in the general population.
Data type representation	Categorical

Indicator name	National survey of heavy episodic drinking
Definition	National surveys of rates of heavy episodic drinking (binge drinking) among adults (aged 15+ years). Heavy episodic drinking/binge drinking is defined as 60+ g of pure alcohol on one occasion, weekly or more often, during the past 12 months.
Data type representation	Categorical

Indicator name	National survey of underage drinkers of alcoholic beverages
Definition	Regular surveys to collect information on alcohol consumption among underage drinkers of alcoholic beverages (children below the legal age for drinking or being sold or served an alcoholic drink) at the national level. This includes school-based and youth health surveys which include but are not limited to the collection of data on alcohol consumption.
Data type representation	Categorical

Indicator name	National survey of young adults
Definition	National surveys of alcohol consumption among young adults (aged 18–25 years).
Data type representation	Categorical

Indicator name	Data on alcohol disseminated in national annual report
Definition	Dissemination of data on alcohol in a national annual report. A national annual report refers to a written report issued on a yearly basis by the government including information and data on alcohol consumption, health or social services utilization, availability of resources for alcohol use disorders, economic aspects or any other important information related to alcohol use.
Data type representation	Categorical

Indicator name	Topics covered in national annual report
Definition	Publication of a national annual report by the government including information and data on the following topics: • underage drinking • drinking among adults • associations with socioeconomic variables • geographical patterns of alcohol consumption • associations with other substance use • the general public's knowledge relating to alcohol • drinking and pregnancy • brief interventions in the primary health care system • alcohol-related hospital admissions/discharge data • alcohol-attributable deaths • drink–driving and alcohol-related traffic accidents • alcohol-related public disorder and crime • expenditure on alcohol-related harm • affordability of alcohol • availability of alcohol • policy response.
Data type representation	Categorical

Indicator name	Report on alcohol-attributable deaths
Definition	Coverage of alcohol-attributable deaths in a regularly published comprehensive report on the alcohol situation in the country.
Data type representation	Categorical

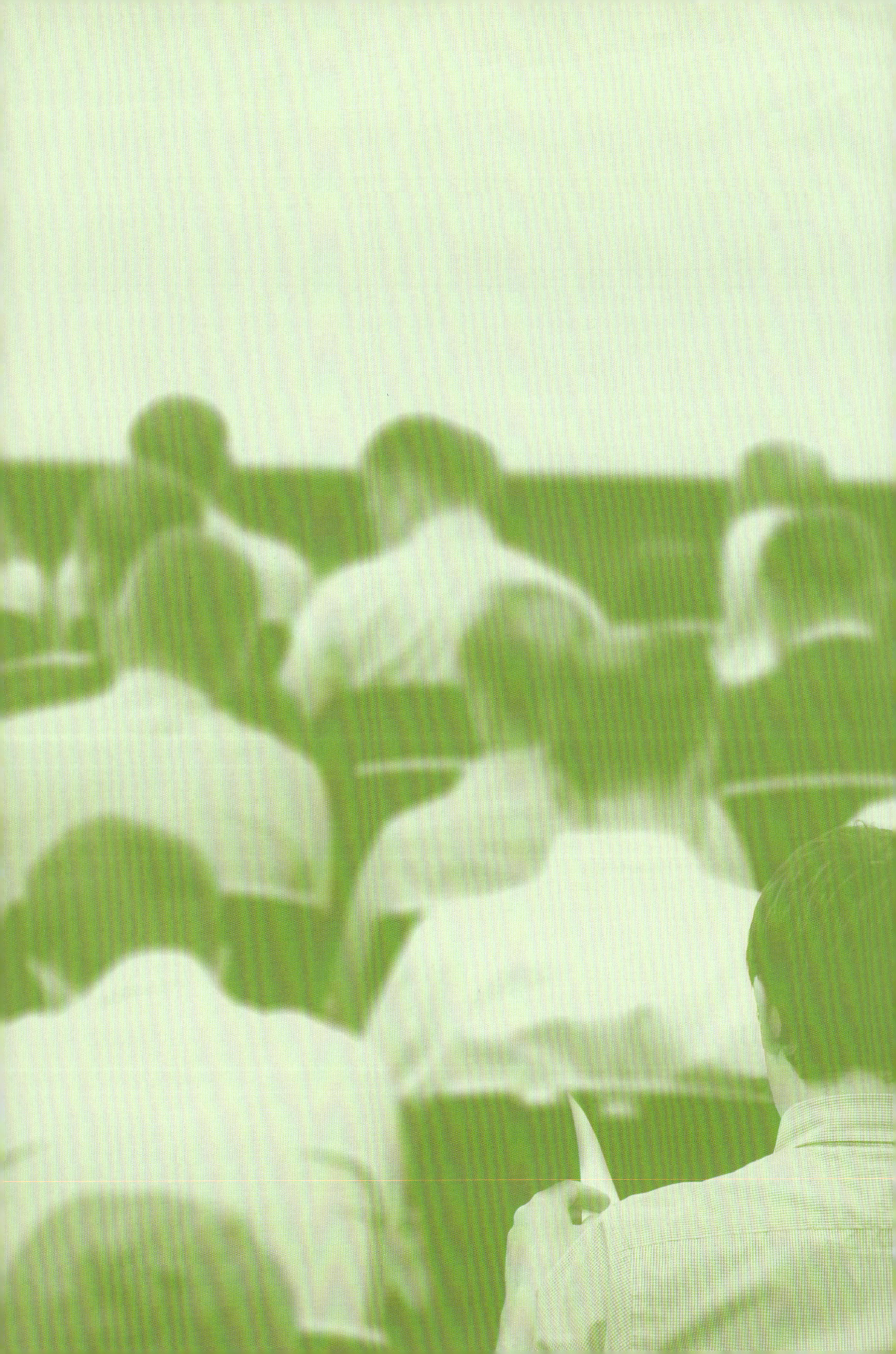

Annex 3
Checklist for policy response

Leadership, awareness and commitment
- Is there a national action plan on the harmful use of alcohol (either stand-alone or as part of another public health plan) that has been reviewed, revised and updated within the last five years?
- Does the national action plan on the harmful use of alcohol or equivalent include measurable outcome and process targets?
- Are there any publicly available health impact assessments on alcohol that regularly monitor the impact of existing and planned policies across a wide range of government departments and sectors?
- Are there coordinating and joined-up mechanisms to ensure policy coherence on the harmful use of alcohol across a wide range of government departments and sectors?
- Is action on the harmful use of alcohol integrated with action on other substances and lifestyles, including physical activity and obesity, mental health and noncommunicable diseases?
- During the previous 10 years, have there been any parliamentary commissions, reviews or reports on alcohol and alcohol-related harm?
- Is there an adequately resourced nongovernmental sector on alcohol?
- Have there been surveys about public knowledge, opinions and attitudes with respect to alcohol? Have these surveys been repeated over time to detect possible changes in opinions and attitudes with respect to alcohol?
- Have surveys been carried out of public views about different alcohol policy measures? Have such surveys been repeated to detect possible changes in views towards different alcohol policy measures?
- Are public funds allocated to alcohol research programmes?
- Are adequate resources provided to government officials responsible for preventing and managing the harmful use of alcohol?
- Have information-based public education campaigns about responsible drinking behaviour and the harmful use of alcohol been implemented and evaluated?

Health services' response
- Are there practice-based and clinical guidelines for early identification and brief advice programmes?
- What percentage of the population is being screened for alcohol use problems?
- What percentage of those identified as having hazardous or harmful alcohol use receive brief advice programmes?
- Are there training programmes for primary care providers on early identification and brief advice interventions? Who conducts early identification and brief advice interventions (for example, family practitioners and/or nurses)?
- Are there systems for monitoring the quantity and quality of early identification and brief advice programmes, so that their effectiveness can be analysed and improved?
- Are there treatment programmes for people with alcohol use disorders and dependence? Are the treatments evidence-based?
- Are there systems for monitoring the quantity and quality of treatment programmes for people with alcohol use disorders and alcohol dependence?
- Is there any financial support for delivering early identification and brief advice programmes? Who receives financial support (for example, health care centres, family practitioners, health care providers)?
- Do midwifery and obstetric services offer pregnant women information and advice about drinking during pregnancy?
- Do social welfare services provide support to family members of individuals with alcohol problems?

Community and workplace action
- Have there been any reviews of existing alcohol education programmes to assess their impact and potential for improvement?
- Have evidence-based guidelines been prepared and disseminated about the role and practice of school-based and public alcohol education?
- Are there any criteria for determining which programmes can be included in school curricula?

- Has there been any review of community alcohol efforts, including recommendations for effective elements and guidance on how to adapt them to the specific needs of the local community?
- Have training programmes been developed to support capacity-building for implementing effective community programmes on the harmful use of alcohol?
- Is there the capacity to evaluate and document community alcohol programmes addressing the harmful use of alcohol, so that lessons can be drawn from experience to strengthen and improve them?
- Has there been any review of workplace programmes on the harmful use of alcohol?
- Is there the capacity to evaluate and document workplace programmes addressing the harmful use of alcohol, so that lessons can be drawn from experience to strengthen and improve them?
- Does current national legislation support and facilitate workplace alcohol initiatives?
- Does current national legislation support and facilitate community initiatives addressing the harmful use of alcohol?

Drink–driving policies and countermeasures
- Are there sufficient data systems in place to monitor drink–driving accidents and fatalities?
- What are the present legal BAC limits for driving? How much public and political sentiment is there for reducing the limit?
- Is it possible to incorporate into regular public opinion polls and surveys some questions on attitudes to drink–driving policies, knowledge of legal BAC limits and drink–driving behaviour?
- Do all driving schools provide information on the risks of drink–driving?
- How are drink–driving laws enforced? Are random breath-testing and sobriety checkpoints used?
- Do the police have adequate resources for effective enforcement? Can fines be used to finance police activity?
- What are the penalties for drink–driving?
- Are the traffic police committed to mounting joint campaigns and activities with national or local authorities to reduce drink–driving?

- Is there an effective road safety transport policy that addresses drink–driving together with road safety measures to reduce the severity and risk of drink–driving accidents?
- Does the health sector have the capacity to deliver brief advice programmes to drink–drivers and treatment for repeat drink–drivers as required by the legislation on driving?
- Are there any public education campaigns on the consequences of being arrested for drink–driving?

Availability of alcohol
- Is there an alcohol licensing system? Are local parts of the system granted sufficient power to decide the density of retail sales and opening hours in response to local issues and potential problems?
- Are there opportunities at a national level for reviewing the days and hours of sale so that they can be adjusted to reduce alcohol-related harm?
- What are the present minimum ages for young people to be sold or served alcoholic beverages? How much public and political sentiment is there for raising the minimum age?
- How is the minimum age enforced?
- If there is a government monopoly on the retail sale of alcohol, is there any threat of disestablishing it? How much public and political support does it enjoy?

Marketing of alcoholic beverages
- Are there any regulatory or co-regulatory frameworks for the content and volume of alcohol marketing?
- Are there regulatory or co-regulatory frameworks for promotion or sponsorship by the alcoholic beverage industry?
- Are there regulatory or co-regulatory frameworks for restricting or banning promotions in connection with activities targeting young people?
- Are there regulatory or co-regulatory frameworks for regulating new forms of alcohol marketing techniques, for instance social media?
- Have there been any reviews or documentation of commercial communications and sponsorship of alcohol including self-regulatory measures by public agencies or independent bodies?

- Are there any effective administrative and deterrence systems for infringements of marketing restrictions?
- Is there any regulation of direct or indirect marketing in some or all media?

Pricing policies
- How has the affordability of alcohol changed over time?
- How feasible is it to tax all alcohol products, for example per gram of alcohol?
- What information is available on the price elasticity of beer, wine and spirits?
- Do existing regulations permit the setting of a minimum price for alcohol?
- To what extent do cross-border issues, or the illegal or informal production of alcohol, constrain tax changes?
- Are there any restrictions on below-cost selling or volume discounts?

Reducing the negative consequences of drinking and alcohol intoxication
- Is there a licensing system for the sale of alcoholic beverages?
- Do licensing authorities have design guidelines for serving establishments that can be used in issuing and renewing licences?
- Are there accredited independent programmes to train servers in their legal responsibilities and in practices that reduce the risk of harm in drinking environments?
- Are there regular efforts to identify establishments associated with greater levels of alcohol-related harm and violence?
- Are the sanctions for violations of licensing laws sufficiently severe, including licence revocation? Does the enforcement body have sufficient resources to perform regular checks? Are enforcement officers sufficiently motivated to do their job?
- Are brief advice and treatment programmes routinely delivered through accident and emergency departments for attendees with alcohol-related injuries?
- Are there any regulations concerning health warnings and product labelling, including alcohol and calorie content (similar to a general labelling used for foodstuffs)?
- Are there clear labelling and warnings concerning alcohol-related harm?

Reducing the public health impact of illicit alcohol and informally produced alcohol
- Is there any information on the size and composition of the market for unrecorded alcohol, including estimates of associated harm?
- Are tax stamps used to indicate when and where duty is paid?

Monitoring and surveillance
- Are routine data on all relevant alcohol-related matters readily available within a reasonable timeframe to monitor the implementation of the action plan?
- Are routine data coherent and compatible with other international data sources and surveys, including those of WHO, the European Commission, the Health Behaviour in School-aged Children Survey and the European School Survey Project on Alcohol and Other Drugs?
- Do existing surveys incorporate the alcohol questions needed to obtain the data required for an annual report on alcohol?
- Are relevant related questions included in all other relevant ongoing surveys?
- Are drinking surveys undertaken at least annually or certainly every two years?
- Do drinking surveys adequately capture disadvantaged and socially excluded groups?
- Are there mechanisms for coordination across relevant government departments to ensure the availability of relevant data?
- Are all WHO and European Commission indicators on alcohol regularly collected and made publicly available?